THE EYES HAVE IT

THE EYES HAVE IT

A Personal View

Christopher Liu

In Support of the Sussex Eye Hospital

To John & Beryl

Best wishes
View
Christopher Liu
28-5-12

Book Guild Publishing
Sussex, England

First published in Great Britain in 2012 by
The Book Guild Ltd
Pavilion View
19 New Road
Brighton, BN1 1UF

Typesetting in Garamond by
YHT Ltd, London

Printed and bound in Spain under the supervision of
MRM Graphics Ltd, Winslow, Bucks

A catalogue record for this book is available from
The British Library.

ISBN 978 1 84624 680 7

To my parents
Paul Saik-Pon Liu
Edith Yee-Bik Li Liu

Contents

Foreword

Ophthalmologists (physicians and surgeons of the eye), like other professionals, long ago acquired a stereotype. They are perceived as exacting perfectionists whose little world is represented literally by the globe of the eye. Their limited horizons are further confirmed by their tendency to sub-specialise in certain parts or functions of the eye: for example, cornea specialists (such as both the author and myself) spend significant parts of their lives absorbed by the complexities of a structure that is just half a millimetre thick. Stereotypes exist to be confounded, however, and this book has been written by an ophthalmologist of distinction who decidedly does not conform to type.

True physician that he is, Christopher Liu is also an excellent surgeon. For years it was one of my privileged duties, as a Consultant at Moorfields Eye Hospital, to train Residents (doctors at Junior and Senior Registrar level) in eye surgery. This was done by the time-honoured master and apprentice, one-to-one principle. All left capable of safely performing the operations in which I specialised (especially corneal transplantation) but their initial aptitude varied widely. A few (and I remember every one) had such natural, innate dexterity and the ability to, as it were, 'think' with their hands while simultaneously observing, reasoning and planning with their eyes and brains, that I often felt honoured to be assisting them; one such was Christopher.

As readers of this book will discover, Christopher rejoices in the exquisite complexity of ophthalmology (a word which means, literally, the science of the eyes). The study of this science is, however, in a purely human sense, far removed from the minor miracles that we are able to perform on an almost daily basis. The restoration of sight, man's principal special sense, is a privilege within our gift and its significance at the interpersonal level has been fully recognised by Christopher, who writes: ' . . . I do not allow anyone in my team to think of the operation as "just another cataract", for it is the eye, sight and life of a fellow human being.'

With remarkable conciseness, Christopher has written the history of the Sussex Eye Hospital, culminating in the celebrations of its 175th anniversary in 2007, and accounts of how we see, the history and current practice of cataract surgery, laser eye surgery, plus an operation to replace the cornea (reserved for those who are blind from corneal scarring) and more besides. He has also assessed the changing fashions in the training of ophthalmologists and the qualities and attitudes that he considers prerequisite for such training. Remarkably, all of this takes place within the context of a frank and honest autobiography. I warmly commend to the reader this arresting, unusual and above all very personal book.

Roger J Buckley FRCS, FRCOphth
Professor of Ocular Medicine, Anglia Ruskin University, Cambridge
Honorary Consultant Ophthalmologist, Moorfields Eye Hospital, London
Honorary Visiting Specialist, Addenbrooke's Hospital, Cambridge

Author's Preface

'Our sight is the most perfect and most delightful of all our senses.'

Joseph Addison (1672–1719)

I have written this potpourri book for a number of reasons. The first question I had was how specialist eye hospitals evolved, particularly the Sussex Eye Hospital where I have worked as a consultant surgeon for fifteen years. I discovered that such eye hospitals are an important part of our heritage, and that they are valuable institutions that work very well. We must therefore support and nurture their continued development and role in our community.

The second question was what led me to become an ophthalmic surgeon in the first place. When examining this, I took the opportunity to record my early years for the benefit of my family. I have compared my own training experiences with those of current trainees and would advocate some return to an apprenticeship system.

Writing this book has allowed me to take stock of the last fifteen years as a consultant, and I now have clear plans for the next fifteen. I hope that all readers will find the book interesting and that it will provide some inspiration to ophthalmologists in training.

This book is divided into three parts.

Part I is an excursion into the history that led to the development of specialist eye hospitals in the early nineteenth century. It covers the early years of the Sussex Eye Hospital, where I now work, and the life not only of its founder, James Pickford, but also of Brighton society that has nourished this remarkable institution for over 175 years. Sadly, detailed records about James Pickford are extremely meagre, though thanks to the help of many archivists across the country we have been fortunate enough to discover fresh, unpublished material. The fragmentary nature of what does exist means that we can give only a few glimpses into events during Pickford's life.

Part II is an account of my early life – background, family, and education – as well as those factors that led me to become an eye surgeon and the exacting but fascinating years of training that were necessary to achieve my goal.

Part III, more detailed and technical, describes how our knowledge of the structure of the eye and our understanding of vision have enabled ophthalmology to advance greatly over the last thirty years. Fundamental scientific discoveries, new machines such as binocular microscopes and sophisticated tools such as lasers, make possible new treatments undreamt of in the past. But all new advances bring fresh challenges. New possibilities generate new demands on the Health Service and on doctors, who both practise their craft and train the next generation.

All royalties from the book, which is dedicated to my parents, will be devoted to the Sussex Eye Hospital's Eyesight Fund and the Sussex Corneal Research Fund. My father, a family physician, was a man of few words, but we followed him by example. My mother supervised our studies but never with undue pressure. My parents made significant sacrifices to ensure that all their children had an excellent education.

I have many other people to thank. First of all, I have been able to draw on the unpublished research conducted by the distinguished international medical historian, Dr June Goodfield. Her interests and writing – along with those of her colleagues, Peter Robinson and Matt Homewood – are now devoted to Sussex history, whether medical or general. They have helped me not only in the research but also in the writing of this book. I am happy to acknowledge my deep debt to them all.

I also thank Professor Roger Buckley for writing the foreword; Professor Harminder Dua for the afterword; my colleague Dr Matt Cooper for support and advice; Lali Moodaley, Sue Cooper and Debbie O'Bryan for proof-reading; Dr Tony Jones for extensive editorial work; Donny Munro; Hugh Williams; Richard Keeler, Curator of the Royal College of Ophthalmologists Museum, for valuable historical information; my colleague Bruce McLeod for inspiring my interest in how specialist eye hospitals came about; Oliver Comyn and Salim Okera.

I owe a special debt to two Brighton residents. First of all, Gloria Wright who provided valuable information on The Brighton Society for the Blind, which was founded in the early nineteenth century and is still flourishing today. Second, Peter Field, Lord Lieutenant of East Sussex and a staunch supporter of the Sussex Eye Hospital, for helping me to understand the wider context of Brighton society.

Finally, I thank my wife Vivienne and our children, Sophia, George and Henry for being wonderfully supportive and understanding during the many months of work on this book.

Part I

1

The Story of Eye Hospitals

Although the word 'eye' is very old, specialist eye hospitals are not, for most were established in the early nineteenth century.

Nevertheless, the treatment of eyes is certainly very ancient. The Ebers papyrus (c.1550 BC) contains over ninety prescriptions for trachoma-related conditions. Roman seals have been found which record the preparation of *collyria* – eye medications – and seals with similar recipes have been found in other countries. One herbal remedy used extensively throughout medieval times, 'eyebright', comes from a native European plant and was so-called because the red and white flowers resembled a bloodshot eye.

Many studies on eyes can be found in the records of the monasteries of Norman Britain, the first treatise on eyes being published in the fourteenth century. Though originally in Latin, an early English translation quickly followed. By the time of Queen Elizabeth some 200 years later much more had been printed, though inevitably not all the recommended remedies were particularly effective. Walter Bayley, the court physician during her reign, had

3

the courage to question the efficacy of urine for bathing the eye, but his alternative suggestion, ale, was not much better!

Bayley – Baley or Baily, his name was spelt in a variety of ways – became Professor of Medicine at Oxford in 1561. Some historians claim that he wrote the first English vernacular work on ophthalmology: 'A briefe treatise touching the preservation of the eie sight, consisting partly in good order of diet, and partly in use of medicines.'

Cataracts – one of my special interests – have been recognised for generations and are still the main cause of blindness throughout the world. In 2009, 17.5 million people were estimated to be suffering from the condition, which occurs when the crystalline lens of the eye becomes opaque and ultimately sight can be severely impaired.

When applied to a defect in the eye, the word 'cataract' has a curious origin. Originally it referred to a waterfall or a portcullis, the gate that drops down in front of a drawbridge or a grating across a window, and was very common in medieval Latin though initially rare in English. Cataract is a figurative use of the word 'portcullis' for even when the eye is open, the cataract obstructs vision as the portcullis does a gateway. Around 1550, we find a French physician, A. Paré, writing about *'cataracte ou coulisse'* – *coulisse* being the French word for portcullis.

The earliest known reference to the treatment of cataracts is over 3500 years old in the Code of Hammurabi, dated 1750 BC. This gives details of 'couching' – the pushing back of the clouded lens by needling with a lancet. The fee payable to the surgeon was specified, so too was the penalty should the patient die or merely lose his sight. In both cases the surgeon's fingers were cut off.

Couching was also practised in Britain and Europe. One

of the best accounts of this treatment comes from the somewhat immodest Richard Banister, who in 1622 wrote; 'in the methodicall practice and cure of blind people, by couching of Cataracts, our English Occulists have alwayes had expeciall care, according to Arts, to couch them within doores, out of the open aire, to prevent further danger.' Interestingly, he included in his book Bayley's earlier work on ophthalmology.

Before modern times the outcome of any medical treatment, whether general or specific to the eyes, was perilous to say the least. Extensive empirical evidence was built up, but the era of experimentation and clinical trials was centuries away. So one treatment was just about as effective as any other. Though by the nineteenth century anatomical knowledge had advanced greatly, very little was known of either physiology or the underlying causes of disease. In his *Ophthalmographia*, published in 1713, Peter Kennedy wrote; 'quacks flourish in all ages, and the eye has always been a happy hunting ground for such practitioners.' Few questioned that quackery, charlatanism and plagiarism were the unenviable hallmarks of ophthalmology in Britain, and some even claimed that this contrasted unfavourably with the clinical approach established in France by more orthodox practitioners.

Yet, ironically, it was connections with France that were to trigger the establishment of specialist eye hospitals in Britain, even though these came about not through peace, but war – predominantly the Napoleonic Wars.

Napoleon first faced the British en masse in Egypt. The battle of Aboukir in 1801 was famous not only for the severity of the fight, but for the occurrence of a severe epidemic during the summer months, caused by Egyptian ophthalmia, an ailment which historians later labelled 'one of the plagues of Egypt.' Army doctors had never seen the disease before; it established itself rapidly and persisted amongst the soldiers for many years. There were soon 160 cases of total blindness in the British forces alone and a further 200 soldiers suffered the loss of one eye. The inflammation was also highly contagious. Assistant Surgeon Power of the 23rd Regiment described it 'the most dreadful disease that has ever visited mankind.'

The rapid onset and spread of the infection is easily explained. Living conditions in towns and villages were highly unsanitary; recurrent plagues of flies rapidly carried infected material around and purulent infections amongst the general population were prevalent. Soldiers living in the dust and sand quickly became infected. Initially the disease was attributed to a combination of factors; arid and burning sand, the heat and blinding glare of the sun and heavy uniforms that suppressed perspiration.

A messy conjunctivitis appeared first, followed by virulent suppuration. Infection spread from one man to the next not only by personal contact, dirty towels and flies, but also through crude methods of treatment.

The actions of the British medical staff were heroic but disastrous. When their physicians observed that the infection usually struck healthy soldiers, logic apparently dictated that to reduce the severity of inflammation, the patient's strength should be drastically reduced. So they were regularly bled through the temporal artery and at least twenty or thirty – at times even sixty – ounces of blood extracted. Meat was forbidden. Drugs such as mercury were administered in huge doses to encourage salivation, along with medicines like antimony that induced vomiting.

The surgeons were kept busy. The diseased conjunctiva – the mucous membrane connecting the inner eyelid and

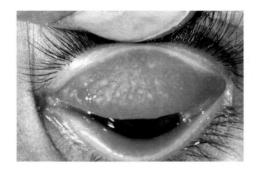

Egyptian ophthalmia (trachoma).
Courtesy of the World Health Organisation.

eyeball – was taken out and the conjunctival blood vessels repeatedly subjected to scarification when superficial incisions were made into the membrane. Since it was thought that counter-irritation methods would be helpful, the patient was blistered on other parts of the body. The effects of the surgery were compounded by the administration of large amounts of powerful drugs such as copper sulphate, lead acetate and silver nitrate. It is surprising that any patient survived, especially since all the procedures were done with filthy instruments.

Logic, no matter how impeccable, can have dire consequences in the absence of good science and so it proved, for the French actually fared much better when treating their soldiers. After the battle on 21st March 1801, Baron Larrey, Napoleon's chief surgeon, attributed the outbreak to heat in the day, cold nights, mists from the lake and heavy fighting. Within 10 weeks the French had treated 3,000 cases and not a single soldier went blind. The French approach was measured; only mild salt washes were applied to the eyes, no powerful drugs were used and only the lightest scarification of the skin on the temple and eyelids permitted.

Both armies took Egyptian ophthalmia back to their own countries and it spread to regiments that had never visited Egypt at all. One surgeon, Edmonston, noted that even though his regiment had been removed to Maidstone, the infection 'raged to a terrible degree'. Within 2 years there were 1,341 cases; there were so many in the 2/12th Foot Brigade that the battalion could not join the Peninsular Campaign and had to remain in Britain. The disease spread from the soldiers to the civilian population and before long, cases had been seen by most medical practitioners across the country.

The severity of the outbreak was so great that the British Army finally took one sensible step. To contain the outbreaks, they decided to concentrate all cases in specific centres. An ophthalmic depot was opened in 1805 at Selsey, near Bognor in Sussex, under the management of a surgeon of the 52nd Regiment, Dr John Vetch. Born in East Lothian, he trained at Edinburgh and later became Principal Medical Officer for Ophthalmic Cases in the Army. Within 6 years, 3,000 cases had been treated in Selsey and Vetch's statistics showed that compared to regimental hospitals, where many soldiers lost their vision completely, only 20 of his patients had to be invalided out for blindness. His success is likely to have been a result of his conviction that transmission of the infection occurred through contact with infected matter from a diseased patient. Not everyone agreed with his theory, but his contemporaries did acknowledge that he was the first to assert this in public and his results were significant.

This, then, was the background to the establishment of eye hospitals in Britain. Soon there was a whole slew – the West of England Eye Infirmary, established in Exeter in 1808; Bristol in 1810; Manchester in 1814 and the Royal Westminster Ophthalmic Hospital in London in 1816. Moorfields, the most famous, was founded in 1805 as The London Dispensary for Curing Diseases of the Eye and Ear. By 1807, Moorfields had become an exclusive, specialised ophthalmic hospital, which they claimed was the first of its kind in the world. Soon ophthalmology was properly established in medical practice and as orthodox specialist practitioners increased in number, quackery slowly vanished and the field went from strength to strength.

There was an additional benefit, for as the success of the specialised eye hospitals became clearly obvious, more and more ophthalmic departments were set up in general hospitals. However, most surgeons were not specialist and it was to be some time before some of their profession would concentrate solely upon eyes.

Though the Sussex Eye Hospital at Brighton was not one of the earliest to be established, it was by no means one of the last. Its founder, James Pickford, had close links with the Army. Connections between Selsey and the Napoleonic Wars are firmly established.

2

The Eye Surgeon in the Nineteenth Century

James Hollins Pickford was born in Bromley, Kent, around 1802. His father, also called James, was an unskilled labourer who later moved to Camden Town with his wife, Frances.

In the early nineteenth century there were usually two ways to qualify as a physician; which path you took depended entirely on your parents' wealth. If they were rich you went to Oxford or Cambridge, and after several years studying Latin and philosophy, but very little science, you would join the practice of a distinguished physician in London or a large provincial town. However, if your parents were poor, you had to obtain an apprenticeship that could be long or short, effective or ineffective, depending on your mentor. But since master surgeons did not usually take apprentices, and when they did, often restricted them to family or friends, the opportunities were few and far between. There was occasionally however a third route.

On 27th April 1824, James Pickford was admitted to the London Hospital as a 'dressing pupil' to Sir William Blizard.

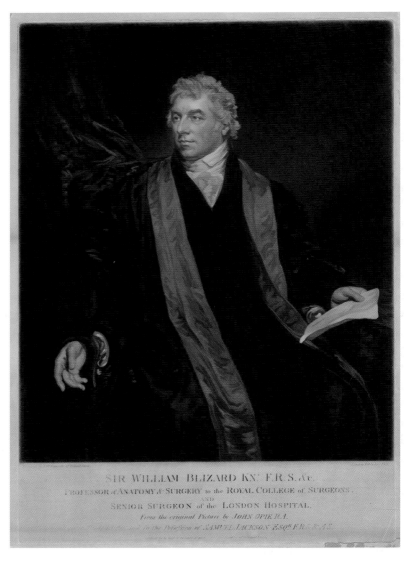

Portrait of Sir William Blizard by Samuel Reynolds.
© National Portrait Gallery, London.

There was a clear-cut distinction between a dressing pupil and an apprentice. A dressing pupil was usually someone who already had some kind of medical experience; it was a common way to gain clinical knowledge, did not take as long as an apprenticeship and was less costly. By contrast an apprenticeship was a legally binding agreement that generally lasted for seven years and cost a great deal more.

A year-long course consisted of attending dressings, operations and daily general practice at Guy's, St Bartholomew's or St Thomas' which between them had 400 beds. For this a pupil had to pay £50 in advance, equivalent to over £1,600 today. Regular lessons in anatomy and surgery cost an additional 12 guineas.

William Blizard also lacked a classical education, so he too had been a dressing pupil articled to Mr Besley, a surgeon and apothecary at Mortlake. Yet his subsequent career was most distinguished. He was elected surgeon to the Magdalene Hospital, London, at an early age. He then persuaded the House Committee of the London Hospital to let him give lectures on anatomy and surgery in two rooms on the east side of the hospital – though he had to pay to have them built himself. These two rooms formed the nucleus of the medical school of the London Hospital. Blizard was so delighted with the two rooms that he commemorated their creation in verse which his friend, Dr Samuel Arnold, set to music. The piece was first performed not in a concert hall but in the London Tavern!

Since there were no organised medical schools at any hospital, the pattern of training was somewhat disjointed. A student might attend lectures in a private home followed by a few hours in the hospital as a walk-in pupil.

Pickford remained with William Blizard a mere twelve months and we have no accounts of his actual training. In truth, our knowledge of the schedule medical students experienced at that time would be very sparse were it not for one lucky fact. In 1791, the Portuguese Minister of Foreign Affairs despatched seven students from Lisbon to London in order to get instructed in their intended profession – surgery. The young men who went to London were not the first to come to Britain from Portugal; one group had already trained in Edinburgh. They might all have gone to France had the French Revolution not been so unpopular with the Portuguese court and these records would never have existed.

The seven young men arrived in October, 1791. The Portuguese *chargé d'affaires* in London, who was told that they would be under his direct supervision, was not overjoyed. However, he found them lodgings and set up a plan of work. They would learn the English language and once they could 'usefully listen to the lectures' they would follow the regular courses of surgery, anatomy and childbirth, and increase their knowledge by attending practical operations in the hospital.

The Portuguese diplomat never ceased to remind his students that they were in his charge. So worried was he that they might fail in their duties since 'the town provides many possibilities of dissipation', he insisted they provide 'proof of their work' by writing a daily journal of the operations they attended, to be submitted every week. When the students protested, the weekly requirement was reduced to a monthly one. But still he kept a very strict eye on them all and records show that there were some unpleasant confrontations.

We know that, at least for a short time, three students fulfilled his orders quite literally to the letter. As Dr Machado de Sousa of the Faculty of Social Science and

Humanities in the New University of Lisbon put it; 'thanks to the strictness of a bad-tempered diplomat' these accounts are unique. True, there are some handwritten text books in the library of St Thomas' in which the British surgeons set out in precise detail how operations ought to be performed but, in contrast, the Portuguese journals contain vivid, minute descriptions of the procedures as they happened and just what they observed. They even made drawings in the journals of prints that were on the wall of the eighteenth-century anatomical theatre in Guy's.

From August to October 1793 their journals describe the extraction of a scirrhous breast and a tumour of the mouth, removal of two cataracts (one of which was 'double'), a hydrocoele (an accumulation of fluid), three amputations (one of the leg, two of the arm), one castration and an attempt to remove a nasal polyp which was not completed because the patient felt the pain was excessive. The surgeons performing these operations were Klein and Chandler of St Thomas', Foster, Lucas, Cooper and Long of St Bartholomew's, and Pickford's teacher, Sir William Blizard, of the London Hospital.

As de Sousa wrote, 'The importance of the journals are not only the interesting technical details, but they show above all, that though these places were not medical universities, the London hospitals took seriously their responsibility not only of treating patients they received, but training their medical staff – a tradition that has not been broken and should always be maintained.'

One can judge from these accounts what James Pickford's own training would have been like.

After leaving the London Hospital, Pickford joined the Army on 19th October 1828, as assistant surgeon in His Majesty's Grenadier Regiment of Footguards, commanded by His Grace, the Duke of Wellington. The regiment had been serving in Portugal the year before, but by the time he joined they had replaced the 3rd battalion in Dublin. While he experienced no fighting, he did develop a great love for Ireland. Lieutenant Colonel Seymour, the present regimental archivist of the Grenadier Guards, believes that this military inactivity is the reason that Pickford would have sought a more interesting position as soon as possible. In July 1829, he resigned. It is possible – though no documentary evidence exists – that during his short time with the 1st Regimental Footguards, he became acquainted with the occupational hazards, medically speaking, of soldiers that led to his abiding interest in eyes.

We know he was in Brighton less than one year later, for on 8th May 1830 he married Anna Henwood at St Nicholas' Church. We are not sure how he spent the intervening time but his obituary mentioned that he studied for 'twelve months in the best hospitals in Paris'. Brighton was originally a poor fishing village, with a population of just 1,000 in 1740. However, by the turn of the nineteenth century, Brighton was a flourishing town of 9,000. There were two factors in the second half of the previous century which stimulated Brighton's growth and appeal. First was the increasing popularity of sea-bathing as a medical cure – a fashion pioneered by Dr Richard Russell, a physician in nearby Lewes, who moved to the seaside so his patients could benefit. The second was a lure that remains universally effective; royal patronage. When the Prince of Wales, aged twenty-one, visited Brighton on 7th September 1783, aristocrats, professionals, fashionable and literary folk soon followed and Brighton's popularity soared. By the time the Sussex County Hospital opened in 1828, the population was 40,000.

But along with the wealthy came a huge number of poor to cater for their lifestyles. So many came seeking work that a medical charity, The Brighthelmstone Dispensary, was founded in 1809. As its president, the Earl of Chichester, rightly remarked:

'... opulence draws round it a circle of poverty; the industrious and the labouring part of the community seeks to dwell where there is the greatest probability of their obtaining employment and support. Where there are many poor, diseases of various kinds and especially epidemics will be of very frequent occurrence, and in such times as these, if disease enter the poor man's habitation, he is at once deprived of the means of subsistence; his circumstances are left to prey upon a mind destitute of resources and the extreme of misery is the consequence... The misery of the lower orders produced by sickness... appeared to be so widely extending, that with all their willingness to relieve and assist, they were convinced that nothing short of a dispensary could meet the exigencies of the case.'

At a meeting in the Bedford Hotel on 22nd August 1832, a decision was taken to establish the Sussex and Brighton Infirmary for Diseases of the Eye. We have no records of who attended, though James Pickford was clearly there since from then on, he is recognised as the founder of what was to become the Sussex Eye Hospital. However, the *Brighton Gazette* in his obituary on 21st January 1875 gives some clues, when they wrote that it was he

'... who first conceived the idea of starting an infirmary for diseases of the eye, which, by the aid of a few

17

friends, he first opened, in one small room in Middle Street. After a time, by his indefatigable exertions, aided by his father-in-law (the late John Mills, Esq.) premises were obtained in Boyce's Street, West Street; a small house, small accommodation for patients (only four beds), and small means. Nothing daunted, however, he still persevered, and, it was mainly owing to his untiring exertions, and the assistance he derived from his personal friends, that at length this small idyllic "charity" was enlarged into what is now one of the most useful and noble of our county institutions, namely The Sussex and Brighton Infirmary for Diseases of the Eye.'

We do know that the hospital was not only for the treatment of eye diseases amongst the rich and the military, which ever since the Napoleonic Wars had maintained strong connections with Brighton. It was also designed to treat eye diseases occurring in the poor. This philosophy has remained a guiding principle at the hospital.

Though Pickford called his new foundation a 'hospital', he actually started in one small room in a house in Middle Street. When, in 1837, larger premises were obtained in Boyce's Street, connecting West and Middle Street, there was accommodation for all of four patients! He complained that their board room was too small and insisted that a wall be pulled down to make it larger. Unfortunately, this wall happened to be supporting the house and, in rectifying the error, costs soared and extra money had to be found.

By 1841 James and his wife, Anna, were living at No.1 Cavendish Place with their four children. Their eldest child, James, became a curate but suffered an aortic

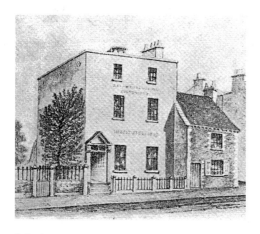

The Brighthelmstone Dispensary in Middle Street, circa 1830.

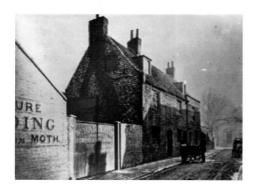

Boyce's Street premises, circa 1870.

aneurysm and died before his father. William Henry, born in 1834, received his MD on 19th February 1858 and followed James into the Grenadier Guards. When William retired on 14th March 1883 he was Brigadier Surgeon. The two daughters never married.

Eventually Pickford felt obliged to improve his medical standing and in 1852, just days after applying, was granted an MD from King's College in Aberdeen, a qualification which today would take many years of study. On 15th April 1852 he appeared before Dr Scott, the Principal of King's College, and Dr Fyfe, sitting with Professors Thomson and Ferguson. On 5th August they reported that they had found the 'following gentleman: James Hollins Pickford of Brighton' duly qualified and recommended for the degree. The archives at King's College do not give details of what questions the examiners asked. Whatever they were, there cannot have been many, for the proceedings were brief and cursory.

Pickford soon became an established and respected figure in Brighton. Even before he sought an MD, he and his wife could afford a maid, a French governess, a cook, a housemaid, a ladies' maid and a footman. Not only did he acquire a whole series of medical honours, including some from Ireland, which he visited regularly, but he also became a Justice of the Peace. He was an ardent amateur archaeologist and took an active part in the preservation of the tomb of Gundreda – the wife of William de Warrenne and daughter of the Conqueror – that was discovered at Southover, Lewes.

He held very strong opinions. On 29th May 1847, *Aris's Gazette,* a Birmingham newspaper, published a letter from him concerning 'the detrimental effects of the inhalation of ether' in which he asserted that 'the annihilation of pain during an operation is hazardous to the patient.' We do not know whether he changed his mind after another, equally strong-minded person who held similarly firm opinions received chloroform during the birth of one of her children. Queen Victoria's patronage of pain relief contributed greatly to the popularity of pain annihilation.

Pickford's expertise was called for on many occasions. On 14th July 1866, an article appeared in the *Hampshire Telegraph and Sussex Chronicle* concerning the 'mysterious death of a lady and suicide of her husband at Brighton', an event that caused 'considerable excitement' in the town! Dr Warder, a physician from Penzance, had been slowly poisoning his wife. He killed her first and then committed suicide. Pickford was called to examine the bodies and gave evidence and, to no-one's surprise, the court ruled that something had been 'administered improperly'.

Pickford had led an interesting and successful life but his lasting legacy was undoubtedly the internationally renowned Sussex Eye Hospital. He remained faithful throughout to its founding principles as one can read in his obituary in the *Brighton Herald*, Saturday 23rd January 1875; 'his advice and services were always at the command of his poorer fellow-townsmen, and by them and by a numerous circle of private friends, his loss will be severely felt.'

3

The Legacy We Inherited

When in 1846 the Sussex and Brighton Infirmary for Diseases of the Eye came under pressure to expand yet again, a purpose-built hospital was erected in Queens Road, next door to the Moon Institute for the Blind. The hospital still has the silver trowel presented to Pickford on his appointment as physician when the first stone was laid on 29th June 1847.

In the meantime a parallel development was occurring which had an equally profound impact on people's lives in Brighton. In 1840 William Moon, a young man studying for the ministry, became blind. He had contracted scarlet fever at the age of four and over the years his sight deteriorated. He was obviously intelligent for he did well at school, though studying was extremely difficult.

By the time he was twenty-one, Moon's sight had gone completely and he became very troubled. However, he came to believe that God had given him the necessary talents for coping with blindness and that he should now utilise these for the benefit of all blind people. Moon started searching for a form of embossed type that people might scan with their fingers, and studied all printing types

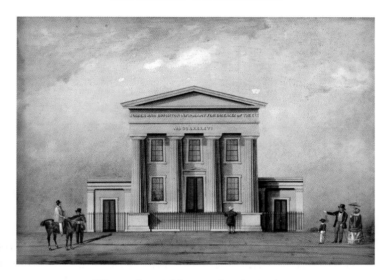

Watercolour of Queens Road premises.

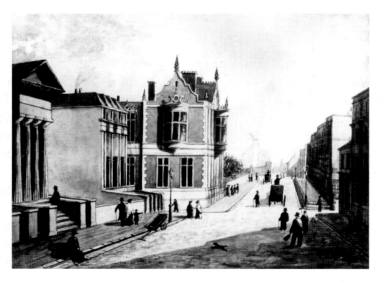

Drawing of Queens Road. The hospital is on the left of the picture.

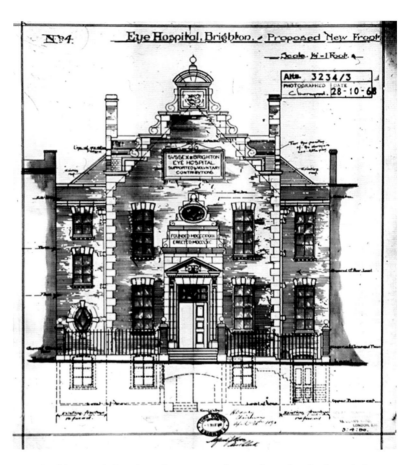

Architectural drawing of a proposed new front for the hospital.

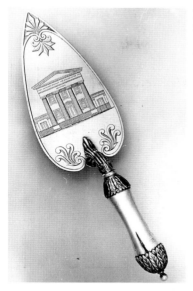

Front of Sussex Eye Hospital silver trowel 1847.

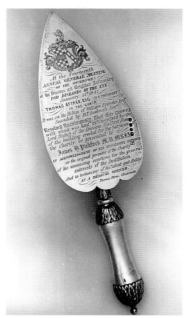

Back of SEH trowel.

25

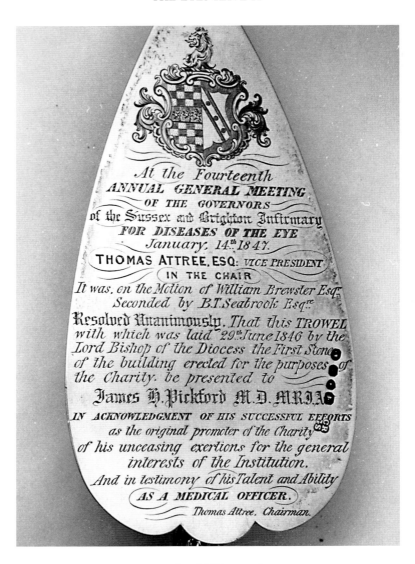

Details of SEH trowel.

then in existence until he found one that really could help blind people to read. This proved easier for children who had sensitive fingers, but very difficult for adults – who accounted for eighty per cent of the blind.

Yet within five years Moon had devised a new embossed type, the forerunner of Braille, which became known as Moon type. Whatever their age or intellectual capacity, a blind person could feel the raised print with his or her fingers and understand the content. Moon's alphabet consisted of nine characters placed in various positions and composed from the simplest geometric forms – a straight line, an acute or right-angled triangle, a circle, a semi-circle. To prevent readers from losing their place, the first line was read from left to right, the second from right to left and a raised curved bracket guided the finger from the end of the line to the one below.

Though now he is mostly remembered for inventing Moon writing, he was actually the pioneer of rehabilitation for the blind, for he helped change their lives. In the early nineteenth century life was terrible for people who had lost their sight; ways of earning a living could be precarious, from busking on corners, to prostitution, to begging – very few could be educated. Moon found this appalling and took action.

He had a small health clinic in his house and set up a school in Eastern Road, Brighton, which eventually became Blatchington Court, then Blatchington Court Trust. As the years went by he invented fresh forms of writing and established remarkable workshops in Queens Road, where Moon books were printed. Besides being an inventor and a humanitarian, he also pioneered educational courses for the blind that led to qualifications. His patients were taught to make brushes, mend chairs, tune

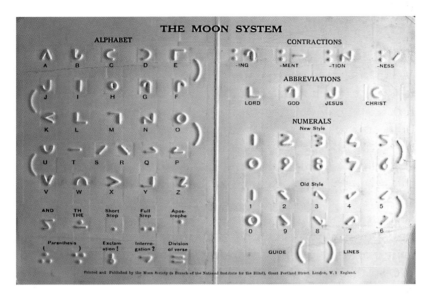

Moon type.

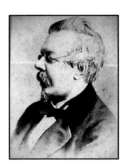

Portrait of William Moon.

pianos and create garments by knitting or sewing. These workshops eventually became the Barclay Workshops that were taken over by Brighton Council.

There were many powerful people backing William Moon and his work, including Sir Charles Lowther, who lost his sight as an infant following an attack of scarlet fever. His mother had imported one of the first embossed books into Britain for him to use. He was a substantial benefactor to William Moon, funding not only the construction of his workrooms, but the initial Moon books and the funded starter packs for individual blind students of all ages who could not afford them.

Internationally, William Moon is most remembered for transposing the Bible into Moon print and then producing it in many different languages. He would take his printing presses by train not only to local places such as Barcombe but also abroad. Accompanied by his son, Robert, who was only sixteen, they delivered a Moon printing press to the Rotterdam Institute for the Blind and stayed for a while to help them set up a printing workshop for Moon writing. Yet since he and his son's activities encompassed support for the poor and a desire to improve their appalling health, they began serious fundraising under the Brighton and Hove Blind Relief Fund, later known as Brighton Society for the Blind. Their activities received wide press coverage.

For fifty years, Moon worked at his system and a vast amount of literature appeared in Moon type, in several foreign languages as well as English and not only the Bible, but educational books, entertaining and scientific, especially astronomical ones. In 1856 he organised the first Home Teaching Society for the Blind, with a circulating library of embossed books. This was such a success that many similar societies were started in other countries.

A few years after World War One, the same situation recurred that Pickford and Moon had faced almost a century earlier. Poverty was still appalling; wounded soldiers were walking the streets; few had any work, and many were homeless. Under the Brighton Society for the Blind, the living legacy of Moon's life work, an appeal was now launched in a local Brighton paper. Money poured in.

* * *

Of course, Pickford's Sussex and Brighton Infirmary for Diseases of the Eye was continuously expanding and soon the existing facilities were once again inadequate for the demands on the service he had started. Finally a new building, costing £40,000, would be erected in Eastern Road, on ground owned by the Royal Sussex County Hospital. An elaborate Masonic ceremony accompanied the laying of the foundation stone in 1933, and two years later on 3rd July, 1935, the hospital was formally opened by Princess Victoria.

Some records of the hospital during the hundred years since it was founded have survived, though they are by no means complete. However, much can be gleaned from the annual reports that have been archived at the Brighton History Centre and the East Sussex Record Office in Lewes. Within them we can find a wealth of detail ranging from patient numbers to rules and regulations to the scale and nature of the diet and the hospital's expenditure. Throughout its entire history right up to the present day, funds have had to be raised for all major alterations. Throughout the nineteenth century, the Earls of Chichester – the owners of Stanmer House, a few miles north of Brighton – helped immeasurably by their own financial contributions, by personal patronage and by twisting their friends' arms.

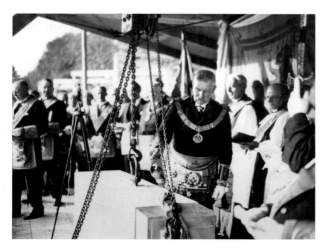

Laying of the foundation stone of the Sussex Eye Hospital, Brighton, by Major R. Lawrence Thornton, CBE, DL, RGD, Right Worshipful Provincial Grand Master. Saturday, 7ᵗʰ October, 1933.

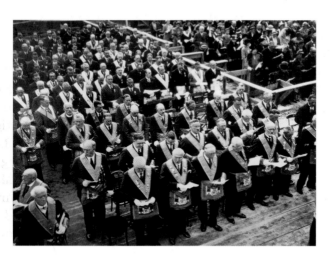

Rare outdoor assembly of Sussex masons. Freemasonry is a fraternity which places great emphasis on a generous heart and charitable giving. They have provided abundantly to the Sussex Eye Hospital over the years, helping with the purchase of new equipment.

THE EYES HAVE IT

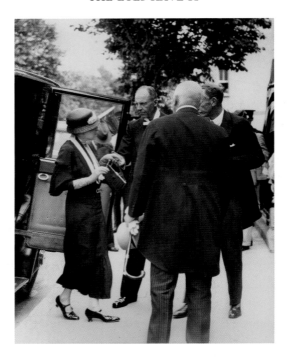

Her Royal Highness the Princess Victoria arriving at the new building at Eastern Road, Brighton, of the Sussex Eye Hospital to perform the opening ceremony.

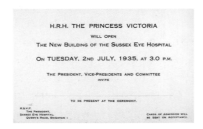

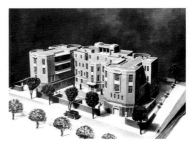

Rear (Sudeley Terrace) view of a model of the Sussex Eye Hospital

These documents also show that providing care for the poor was a constant objective. For example, in the annual report of January 1909 we find the rules under which patients could be admitted. The first states: 'the hospital should be opened with the approval of the Committee of Management, for the reception of the INDIGENT POOR labouring under diseases of the Eye, every week day at 12 o'clock and on Sundays for casualties only.'

Another rule specified that 'patients, when discharged, shall return thanks to Almighty God at their respective places of worship for the benefits they have received, and also the governors who recommended them', though one wonders how this was enforced!

However, annual reports are a somewhat formal way to appreciate and understand the lives of those involved in all aspects of the hospital. There are other sources, such as reminiscences and journalistic accounts, and one especially is both enlightening and enchanting.

When in 1930, the hospital was yet again in the throes of fundraising, the *Nursing Mirror and Midwives Journal* sent a lively reporter down to cover the story. The article is signed with initials only – 'EMP' – and begins with noting that the hospital has 'in its curious planning' much to please and interest the student of history. However, from the nursing point of view the hospital was nothing like so pleasing, being, to say the least, full of practical disadvantages. The matron, Miss L. Goulding, agreed with the journalist's analogy with Lewis Carroll's famous work:

'Indeed, the whole hospital reminded me irresistibly of Alice in her elongated state after she had nibbled the wrong side of the mushroom – an impression which was strengthened when I had been round with Miss

Goulding on a tour of inspection. The building is immensely tall and narrow – there seems to be but one really good-sized room on each floor – and the amount of valuable space wastefully occupied by a winding staircase from the entrance hall and other minor staircases is truly deplorable.'

EMP was next taken on a tour through the Outpatients Department, the comfortable waiting hall, the up-to-date consulting rooms, the dark rooms and the well-equipped operating theatre tiled in green and white. He learned that in 1929 there had been 13,000 outpatient attendances and 500 inpatients, with one ward for men and another for women. Matron was at pains to point out that the interior was to be completely re-worked; the number of beds would be increased with additional wards for septic cases, private cases and children.

The journalist commented that each ward had a pleasant 'old-world atmosphere with green walls, pink counterpanes and quaint antique chairs of polished wood with long, sloping backs'. The writer also noted that 'from the ward windows it is possible to see the sea from a little distance away, and from the women's ward a flight of tiny stairs leads up into a little turret chamber, which is used as a day room by patients who are able to be up.'

Everyone was proud of their most up-to-date feature – a wireless in each ward, an inestimable boon for patients with eye problems.

Next on the tour were the nurses' dining room and the self-contained flat where the staff lived. Miss Goulding had two sisters, two assistant nurses and four probationers under her care. Though all their meals were taken over at the hospital, there was a tiny kitchen with a gas stove so they could make themselves hot drinks before going to bed. Probationers were taken in at the age of seventeen and a half but only if, as Matron insisted, they were 'of the right type' and preferably with a secondary school education. Their salary was £24 in the first year and £26 in the second. Once qualified as an assistant nurse, they received £40. All were given the fabric for their uniforms, but had to make them up themselves.

EMP next met Mr Neville, who was organising the grand historical pageant and fete that would take place the following month in aid of the rebuilding fund, whose patron was Princess Mary, the only daughter of King George V and Queen Mary.

However, EMP was somewhat taken aback when Mr Neville told him that the event would occupy 3 whole days, 3,000 participants would attend and that 'The French ambassador has promised to perform the opening ceremony, and, in addition to nearly one hundred stalls and sideshows, we are having great attractions of an historical pageant, that includes the entry of Jeanne d'Arc into Orleans and the coronation of Napoleon in Notre Dame.'

While the participation of the French is in itself somewhat bewildering, their choice of tableau for the pageants is even more so. Did they mean to remind the noble burghers of Brighton of the origin of eye hospitals through the Napoleonic Wars? Whether the French themselves made a donation to the rebuilding costs of such a substantial size that it merited an invitation to their ambassador to perform the opening ceremony, we still do not know.

Further reminiscences written sixteen years later, in the years after World War Two, give details of the consultants, matrons, sisters and nurses, and exact accounts of just what patients undergoing cataract surgery had to endure.

The admission procedure 'was lengthy for there were many details to check'; they had to be reminded how important it was to keep absolutely still during their post-operative period. The patients' eyes would be padded for at least twenty-four hours; Sonalgin, a hypnotic drug, was given for the first two nights; the nurses had to feed them and only their hands and the skin around the mouth were washed. For several post-operative nights their hands were tied; a cuff was put around each wrist with a crepe bandage tied over it and fastened to the bedstead to prevent them touching their operated eye. Not surprisingly, the combination of having their eyes covered and being tied down caused great confusion in many patients. Dark glasses were worn on days three and four during daylight hours, though the operated eyes were still covered at night. On the fifth day the patient was allowed up, but with strict instructions neither to bend forward, nor sneeze, nor cough. Finally, after ten traumatic days, they were allowed to go home.

This was the protocol for cataract patients. Those with a detached retina had to withstand even longer periods of immobility, being completely flat for a week and generally confined to bed for another two or three weeks, with both eyes doubly padded.

The paper reveals that in the late 1940s there were over 100 outpatients each afternoon, but since there was no appointments system, most turned up around 1.30 p.m. and the last did not leave until after 5.00 p.m.

Life for the nurses in this post-war period was still very restricted. Lights had to be out at 10 p.m. and the night sister would personally enforce this rule. There were no keys to any bedroom doors. Their board and lodging was free, uniform and personal clothes were also washed free of charge, and local chemists gave them a discount of one penny on every twelve spent. But food was rationed and even that available in cafés was very limited, so there was very little on which to spend their annual salary of forty pounds!

Part II

4

My Early Years

I come from a strong medical background. There were many doctors in my family which though ethnically Chinese, lived in Burma (now Myanmar). My grandfather was a carpenter, whose first wife died. He remarried and, as was common in those days, had many children, two of whom became doctors. My father, Paul Saik-Pon (Liu), their ninth child, was the youngest but by the time he was to go to medical school his father had died. Fortunately, he had two wonderful elder brothers who stepped in to help.

My Uncle Saik-Ying had studied at Edinburgh, specialised in respiratory diseases and was medical director of a hospital in Rangoon (now Yangon). However, though Burma was rich in resources, the country was very badly run, so not only he but also most of my cousins emigrated to America. My other uncle, Saik-Chung, was in charge of the Burmese inland waterways, including the Irrawaddy, and became hugely influential. When, having married into their family, my mother arrived in Rangoon for her first visit, my uncles not only asked the air traffic controller to send a message to the plane, but were also on the tarmac to welcome her – as if she were royalty on a state visit!

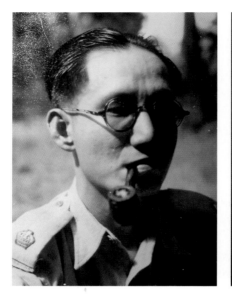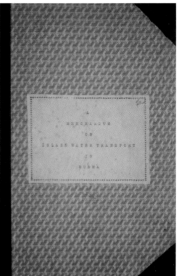

Uncle Saik-Chung and his report 'A Memorandum on
Inland Water Transport in Burma'.

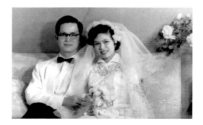

Wedding photo of my parents.

I never met Uncle Saik-Chung since he died in a car crash the year before I was born. But both uncles were indirectly most important to me, since they supported my father through his medical education. They decided he would train in Hong Kong. Once he qualified he became a general practitioner, met my mother, Edith Yee-Bik Li, and settled down happily.

My mother came from a very old Hong Kong family, also with medical connections. The Li family were distinguished and successful, both economically and politically, and still are. They remained in Hong Kong during World War Two, when it was occupied by the Japanese. My mother still remembers the massacres.

Sadly, her father too died young and whereas traditionally the brothers would assume responsibility for the children – as my uncles did for my father, and my father was to do for some of my cousins – in some families the surviving brothers would often snatch their entitlement. So even though my grandmother's family was very wealthy, with a wide portfolio of shares in various companies, she experienced great difficulty in bringing up her nine children and over the next twenty years pawned family jewellery to raise funds.

The Li family was nevertheless a great inspiration to me. They are somewhat like the Rothschilds, some branches were rich, others not at all. But their qualities embodied the vigour with which the whole family raised their children. Through their strong belief in education and the opportunities it provided they eventually assumed key positions in society, from Chief Justice to company directors, owners of banks and professors of surgery and music. They provided me with a role model regarding the importance of learning, of working hard and getting to the

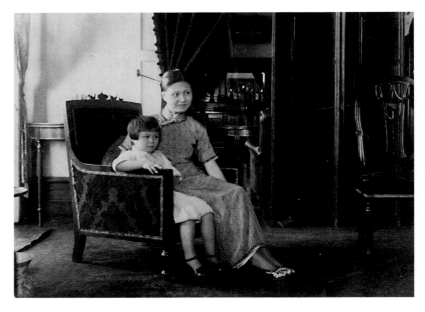

My mother as a child seated with her mother.

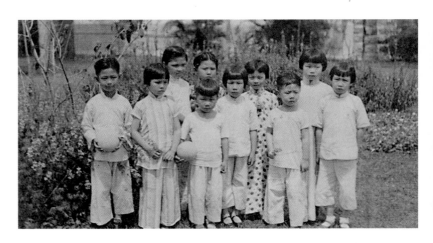

My mother (second from the left) as a child and some of her siblings and cousins.

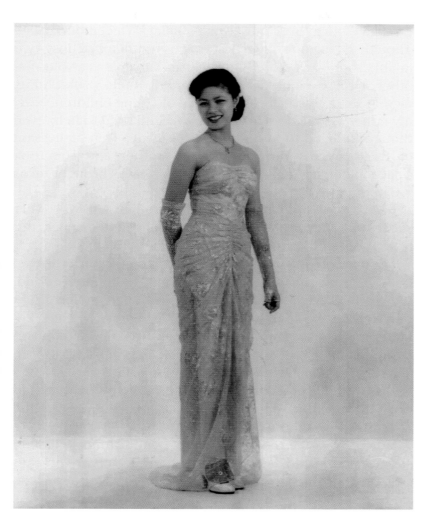

My mother when crowned Miss Hong Kong in 1952.

top of one's profession, of philanthropy and being generous with one's time and money.

I was born in Hong Kong on 9th December 1959. Though I had one older sister, my mother had lost two infants the year before. One was just over a year old, the other a mere eight days. My second uncle, Saik-Chung, died in a car crash leaving a family of young children. Now my father assumed their father's role and tried to help even though he lived thousands of miles away. This succession of tragic events traumatised my mother and she took solace in converting to Catholicism, so I was brought up as a Catholic.

I have two surviving siblings: a brother who is a very successful lawyer and a sister who became a teacher, but retired on medical grounds with severe epilepsy.

My first school was St Teresa's Kindergarten, a mixed Catholic nursery in Kowloon, Hong Kong; my second, their primary school at the same site. Then, when I was nine or ten, I joined my younger brother at La Salle Primary, a Catholic school for boys, and then moved on to their secondary school La Salle College (both also in Kowloon). The Order of the De La Salle Brothers was founded by a French priest in the seventeenth century and their schools and universities are to be found in eighty countries throughout the world.

When I was the tender age of five, my parents decided I should start piano lessons. But, according to my brother and sister's piano teacher, I was already too old to start! So my mother sent me to art classes instead. When I was thirteen, I started to paint quite differently. Everything was in high contrast; I no longer bothered to blend the borders, or paint gradations, whether in colour or texture. Yet although all my brush strokes were very bold they

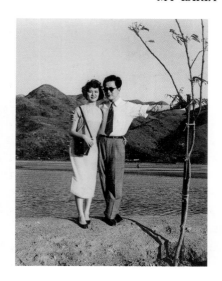

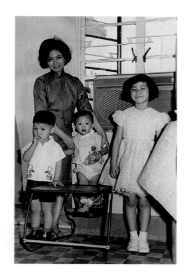

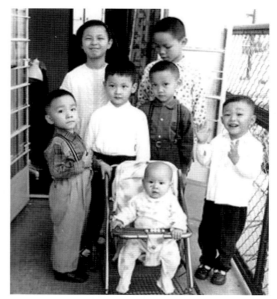

Old family photographs.

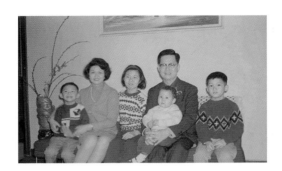

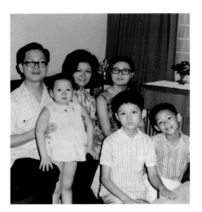

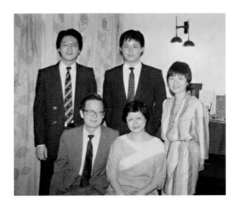

Old family photographs.

appeared blended, blurred into something which I thought was lovely and natural looking.

I had not deliberately changed my style of painting; I had become short-sighted. This was discovered not because I was unable to see the blackboard at school, or watch television, for somehow I just managed these, but through my painting. I realised I had a problem with my eyes and it was there and then that I decided to become an eye surgeon.

By that time my career was more or less decided, for children quite often follow in their parents' footsteps. So since on all sides we were a medical family, my natural aspiration – my vocation – was to become a doctor, but what sort of a doctor? Here my eye defect motivated me. I knew enough science to know that short sight tended to lead to screwing up your eyes in order to see clearly, basically because you are deliberately narrowing your eyelids to a slit. Then it acts like a pinhole and by reducing the aperture and so increasing the depth of focus, sharpens sight.

Having to wear glasses was a hateful impediment. I knew my condition could only worsen and was wondering how it would end. Would the glasses just get thicker and thicker? Would my life just be a big blur? I was determined to cure this problem.

I decided to continue my education in England, which held a great attraction for me, though I have to admit that this came from watching films showing picturesque country houses and excellent boarding schools. I was too young to consider the climate! I just wanted to go somewhere exciting.

However, there were several obstacles. The first was finance. The second was my age, since I was only fourteen,

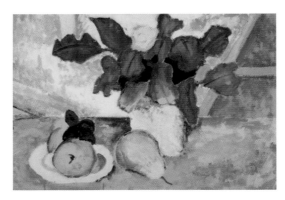

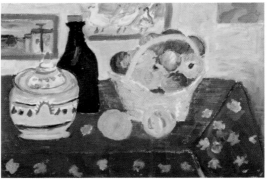

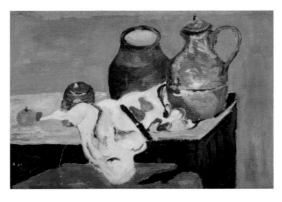

The author's renditions of Cézanne paintings when he was aged eleven, before he became shortsighted.

but my scholastic achievements proved a much more serious impediment. Up to that point I had not worked very hard and my examination results in those subjects I did not like were dire. So I promised that if I was allowed to go to England I would start afresh, work very hard and force myself to tackle things I disliked.

Fortunately, several factors were working in my favour. Other boys at La Salle College were seeking education abroad and on the recommendation of Brother Michael, our careers master, several of us went to Prior Park College, Bath, a school then run by an Irish order of Christian Brothers. It wasn't so much a recommendation as a command; he said, 'You will all go to Prior Park' – and we did!

My parents decided to accompany me to my new school. Even though my father would fly regularly to see his family in Rangoon, air travel was not at all usual – at least not in Hong Kong – and this was only my second flight. The aeroplane was a small Boeing 707 and extremely cramped. The journey took twenty-four hours with one stop in India, another in the Middle East and a third in Rome, before arriving in London.

Just over thirty years ago and aged fifteen, I arrived in England and joined the Lower Fifth Form at Prior Park, with no fewer than seven other boys from Hong Kong. I remember Brother Power, the President (Headmaster), and Brother Coleman who was always to the point, and rather fierce. Though Brother (now Father) Jack Keegan was very kind by the time I arrived, I understand he had mellowed! Brother Miller, who introduced us to Chaucer, did not mind foreign boys not doing well in his classes, but he was almost tearful when English boys took no notice of English literature! Brother Delaney and Brother Cainen helped run the St Paul's House (the senior boarding house), and were

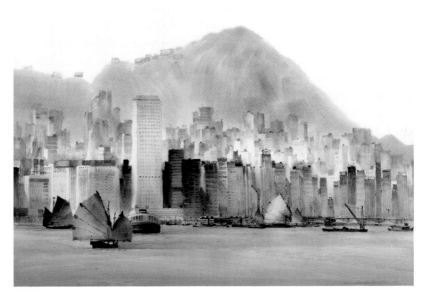

Watercolour of the Victoria Harbour, Hong Kong, in the 1970s. The 52-storey Connaught Centre (now Jardine House) still stands. When completed in 1972, it was the tallest building in Hong Kong and Asia.

so alike that it took me a while to work out that they were two different people. When I saw one in the Study Hall and then, immediately afterwards, he appeared somewhere else, I thought the brothers had supernatural powers. When both finally appeared together, I was in total shock!

There were inevitable problems. Bullying was rife, but most teachers were very kind. I was protected by Brothers Joe Cainen and Jack Keegan, who helped me with music and my tasks for the Duke of Edinburgh Gold Award.

Ironically, having made the decision to work extremely hard, I found there were many boys in my year who were even lazier than I had been before my transformation. Since my academic work went well and I left many of my contemporaries behind, I was labelled a swot and so had a difficult social life. In any case, looking different from everyone else, and not being able to speak English properly, attracted all kinds of unpleasantness.

However, some things were certainly easier. Those of us who came from Hong Kong had a far stronger grounding in science and maths than our British contemporaries. But though I forged way ahead in those fields, I never caught up in subjects such as Latin where others had already done two or three years. My saving grace was a facility with French.

My reliance on glasses was the reason I decided to become an eye doctor, yet on one occasion I could easily have lost my sight altogether. One weekend I decided to see what would happen when concentrated sulphuric acid was mixed with concentrated sodium hydroxide, and created some significant fumes in an explosion in Vic Ferguson's biology lab. I was lucky to have survived this unsupervised experiment at all.

On reflection, my stay at Prior Park was a somewhat

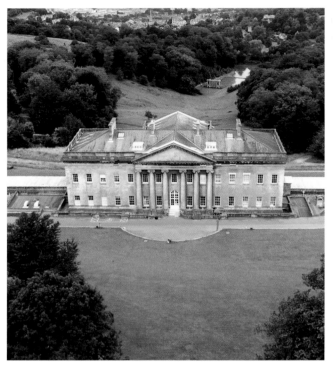

The Mansion of Prior Park College with the Palladian Bridge in distant view.

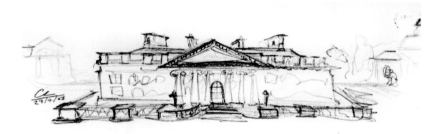

The author's pencil drawing of the Mansion – a mug design for Prior Park Association (alumni society).

confusing time, for we had to speak only English – a new experience for me – and even when I could speak it reasonably well, people still could not understand me. If we Chinese boys were caught speaking Chinese amongst ourselves, or the Central and South American or Gibraltarian boys speaking Spanish, there was real trouble.

What made matters even more confusing was that all Westerners looked the same to me, with large eyes in various shades of blue or hazel, pointed noses and pale skin.

Prior Park College was beautiful; a Palladian Grade I listed building, up on the hillside with stunning views of the town – I loved it. This was also the first time I had to mix with people of other cultures. Britain has now embraced multiculturalism. My personal feeling is that it is good to keep one's culture, so as to keep one's identity. However, segregation is harmful and tolerance and forgiveness are the keys to a harmonious world.

5

From Apprentice to Consultant

I remained at Prior Park for four years, though I managed to return home every summer. I kept my resolve, studied hard and did extremely well in both my 'O' and 'A' levels. I also achieved Grade 8 Classical Guitar and the Duke of Edinburgh Gold Award, as well as significant achievements in the Combined Cadet Force. I was disappointed not to have got into Cambridge. I had applied to Clare College, but without success and even though I was placed on the waiting list, no other college picked me up.

Fortunately, I received an offer from Charing Cross Hospital Medical School in London. Looking back, you cannot always recall what influenced career choices, but I do remember that I liked their brochure very much, with its dazzling black and white photograph of the new lecture theatre. I was interviewed and offered a place and so began my studies at one of the most famous schools in the history of British medicine.

The medical school was once in central London, but by the time I started in 1979 it had moved out to Hammersmith. Going from a Grade I listed building in Bath, with acres of grounds and superb views, to a run-down inner-city area, as Hammersmith was in those days, was a considerable shock. Notting Hill, where I lived in the halls of residence during my first year, bore no comparison to the elegant and sought-after area we see today.

Two years of preclinical studies were followed by three years of clinical work. However, since I had done well in the first two, I was allowed to take an extra year and take a BSc honours degree.

In my sixth and final year, part of my student elective was taken at the famous Moorfields Eye Hospital in the City of London. Since this only lasted for a fortnight, I just followed the professors around and asked questions. Luckily an uncle of a friend introduced me to other people, all several years my senior but all most helpful. I also met Dr Seah Lay Leng – now the chief oculoplastic surgeon at the Singapore National Eye Centre – who gave me significant guidance when I was climbing the professional ladder. Not only had I studied ophthalmology extensively as an undergraduate, well beyond the norm for most students, but I was confident of my ability and I was delighted to receive the undergraduate prize and a commendation for the national Duke-Elder Prize, both in ophthalmology.

Once I was qualified, in July 1985, house jobs followed, generally six months medical work and six months surgical. My first period as houseman was also at Charing Cross and consisted of three months with a respirologist, Professor Abraham Guz, followed by two with a geriatrician, Dr Ivan Walton. Professor Guz was a quintessentially absent-minded professor. Legend has it that one day he parked at a newsagents but then took the tube home, leaving his car outside the shop with his children still inside! He also tended to chew his tie. On one formal occasion the Professor of Surgery, who was sitting next to him, deliberately dangled his tie close to Guz. Naturally, Abe started to chew and never understood why the entire audience was rocking with laughter.

Absent minded or not, he ran a large and highly efficient team and to be his houseman was very prestigious. There were weekly 'grand rounds' and each had a medical case and a surgical case. I was by far the lowliest and youngest person present and it was my personal responsibility to file all the clinical results in the patients' records. Once I failed to do this and as Abe did not have access to the latest figures at the very moment he needed them, he sacked me on the spot. Thankfully, the ward clerk helped me file the data later and I was reinstated!

Bad news from home caused a sudden interruption in my career plans. My father developed cancer, though my mother did not tell me until my final examinations were over. When he became terminally ill I decided to return home. So my second house job, which began on 1st January 1986, was in Hong Kong's New Territories at the Prince of Wales Hospital in Shatin, where there was a new medical school with an efficient clinical side. The job was highly pressurised; when I was on call I was working two nights in three, as well as all day, and looking after thirteen wards with hundreds of patients.

After six months I became an anatomy lecturer at the Chinese University of Hong Kong – all part of my preparation for a surgical career. In fact I had already mapped out my career path and I have now taken most of the steps I wrote down on a filing card when I was a medical student.

By December 1986, when my father's condition had stabilised, I was back again at Charing Cross Hospital as senior house officer in the Ophthalmology Department, where I stayed for about sixteen months. Sadly, my father passed away soon after my return to Britain.

My ambition was to have further training at Moorfields, but positions there were already hugely competitive. I had two alternatives; I could do a period of research, publish some papers and get a master's degree or a doctorate, or I could do a second period of being senior house officer at a feeder hospital. Indeed I was given a chance to work on laser refractive surgery at St Thomas' Hospital, but Tim Leonard, a consultant ophthalmologist and my then boss and mentor, advised me against taking that route. The field was so new, he said, that one couldn't possibly predict the outcome. If only I had known.

Nevertheless, Tim did make a valuable suggestion: I should go to the Western Ophthalmic Hospital (now Western Eye Hospital) in Marylebone Road. The Western was a springboard into Moorfields in the same way that certain prep schools are into some of the best public schools. They had very good people and excellent teaching and surgical programmes, and since the place was always busy the experience to be gained from seeing huge numbers of patients would be invaluable. I took his advice and my whole time there was very demanding. I remember one morning in casualty when I saw fifty-two patients, did two minor operations and one split skin graft that involved harvesting skin from behind the patient's ear. My patient had a skin lesion near their lower eyelid, which I removed, closing the wound with skin I had just harvested.

I was still not a fully-qualified ophthalmic surgeon. As I had earned the consultants' trust I did have my own operating list fairly early on, though, of course, I was watched very closely. My interest in ophthalmology had begun so early that I already had a high degree of training

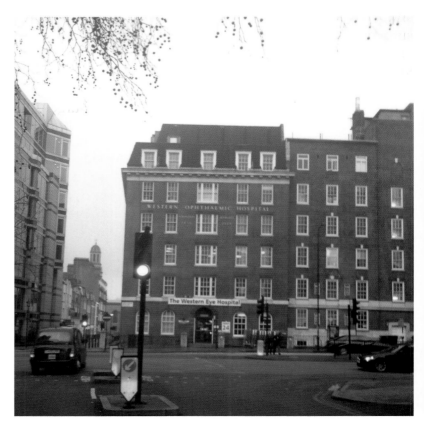

The Western Ophthalmic Hospital, affectionately known as the Western.

and I was actually very dextrous – a blessed gift for a surgeon. Whether this came about from years of using chopsticks, or because I play the classical guitar, I don't know! What I do know is that if I can see how a procedure is done, I can replicate it without instruction. Admittedly, the level of dexterity demanded from an eye surgeon is several degrees more sophisticated than that required when eating grains of rice with chopsticks. Moreover, it is true that all forms of surgery demand the same sort of skill. Although things in ophthalmology are on a much smaller scale and require a high degree of precision, all quality workmanship is similarly demanding.

In addition to my early interest and dexterity, I regularly watched training videos. So even before I was fully qualified as a doctor I knew all the steps for cataract surgery as practised at that time. All this meant I had a precocious surgical career throughout my post-graduate training.

* * *

I remember three key surgical experiences very clearly indeed. My first cataract operation in 1987 at Charing Cross Hospital marked the very first occasion of cutting into an eye.

The second memorable occasion circa 1990 was during my time at Moorfields, when I made a controlled tear for a cataract to pop out. I was making a continuous circular opening in the lens anterior capsule – not destructively, but as part of the procedure. I remember an amazed Mr Hungerford, an eye cancer specialist, going into the operating theatre next door to tell his colleagues what a trainee had just done. But I found that I could naturally visualise three-dimensional spaces within the eye and how to manipulate the situation in order to complete a particular manoeuvre.

The third memorable occasion was when I operated on my first private patient in 1996. This may sound odd, but all my previous operations had been done as part of my NHS work, so to know that I was actually being paid for that specific procedure felt strange.

* * *

The next step on the professional ladder was becoming a Registrar at Moorfields. I was there for three and a half years from 1989 to 1992, and soon found that their professional structure was quite different from other eye hospitals. The trainees were placed at two levels; Registrars and Senior Registrars. They both did the same things, but were attached to different consultants and the rank was clearly different. Once again, it was a little like a public school. There was a clear hierarchy of an Upper House consisting of Senior Registrars and a Lower House of Registrars. When I applied to get into the Upper House, I was not successful even though I tried very hard indeed.

Though the Moorfields' appointment procedures were mainly internal, they did start a tradition of taking in people from the outside. This was extremely sensible, for competition to get to and stay at Moorfields was relentless and the authorities were clearly concerned about too much 'in-breeding'. So people who had been in Senior Registrar positions elsewhere in the country were often appointed for a year and placed in a third category – Fellows. Though above the Senior Registrars in the hierarchy, they were expected to be collegial with them. Yet as every single trainee was competing for the same surgical experience, the Fellows at the top often got the most interesting cases.

Eventually, people were grumbling; you go to

Moorfields, do a hard slog but don't even get promoted! So the wisest strategy was to get training elsewhere, become highly proficient, then go to Moorfields as a Fellow and get all the best opportunities.

Though I never made the Upper House, I met some really inspirational people at Moorfields. Mr John Hungerford was one such. He might have been grumpy at times but he taught me a great deal about eye tumours. Ophthalmology is mostly about improving the quality of life, but when it comes to ocular tumours, death can intervene. He taught me to be serious about such things and led by example with his own solemn approach, reflected in the dark suits and dark ties that he always wore.

Amongst others from whom I learnt much were Peter Wright, a brilliant specialist on corneal inflammatory diseases; Roger Buckley, who was very knowledgeable about contact lenses, corneal grafting and allergic eye diseases and John Lee, a world-renowned squint specialist. John, an Irishman from a family of eleven siblings, was formidable. You never really had to talk to him because he would ask questions and then answer them himself. He could do all the crosswords, knew all the classics and was a very clear thinker. I believed he knew everything! Both Peter Wright and John Lee have served as President of the Royal College of Ophthalmologists.

So it was my great fortune to be involved with very special people, of exceedingly high calibre, in a traditional system of one man and his dog; the Senior Registrar or Registrar serving and learning from one consultant. The team of two (or three if there was also a Fellow attached to the firm) would work very closely together, as in an old-fashioned apprenticeship during which the trainees soon learned that medicine was not just about facts, but

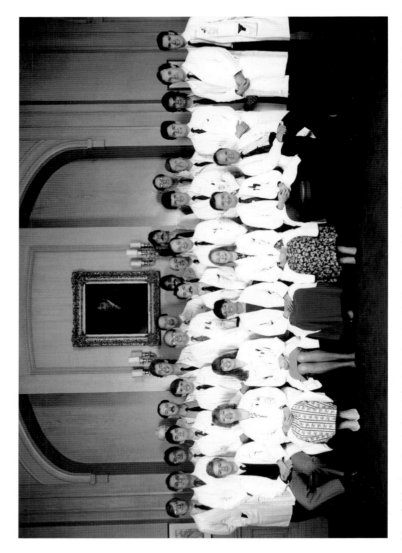

Moorfields Eye Hospital Residents Spring 1991. Courtesy of Mr Keith Barton MD, FRCS, FRCOphth, FRCP.

attitude. The whole essence of being a doctor is how best to help your patients; this involves much more than being a clever technician with instruments. Another element that I was imbibing was the importance of training the next generation.

Such attitudes were familiar to me. I had learnt them, not so much by talking to my father, because he was working most of the time, but by seeing many examples of his superb, holistic care.

* * *

When in 1992 I moved on to become a Senior Registrar at Addenbrooke's Hospital in Cambridge, I was delighted. God had given me a second chance to go to Cambridge and this time my application had been successful.

I had worked so hard at Moorfields that once in Cambridge, I felt I had been released into paradise. The town was beautiful; there were the joys of the River Cam, of undergraduate life, of working with a world-famous ophthalmologist, Peter Watson, who in certain respects I have copied. I learnt so many things there, particularly how to make a small incision for keyhole cataract surgery.

I began research on suturing techniques, working with Chris Hammond, to discover what kind of knot, granny or reef, and in what formation, gave the most compact knot with the smallest volume. If you tie large knots in the cornea when you come to take them out you have to pull hard, which is the last thing you want to do. We found that a 2.1.1 granny knot – tying one loop one way, the second another way and the third the first way again – was the most compact and our results were published in the *British Journal of Ophthalmology*.

I rented a house from one of the consultants and since

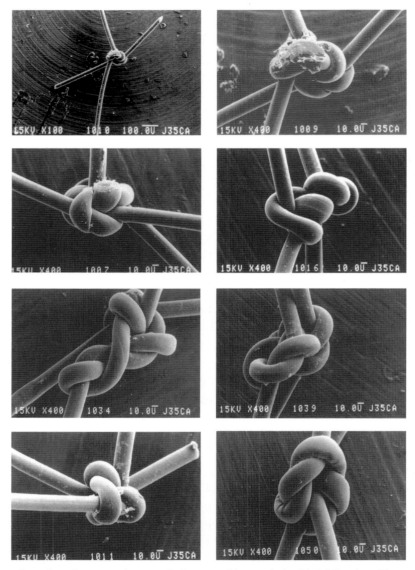

Scanning electron microscopic images of knots tied with 10-0 nylon. The suture material is thinner than human hair. Reproduced from the *British Journal of Ophthalmology*.

this was in an area amongst all the undergraduates, I mixed with them too. My house wasn't very big, but I was paying the entire rent myself. When another doctor, Mahmoud Soliman from Egypt, needed accommodation we decided to share expenses. He was a Fellow to another consultant at Addenbrooke's and is now a professor in Cairo. It was through him that I met Vivienne.

One day he said, 'Christopher, I have found your future wife.' I didn't take him at all seriously, for at that time I was greatly attracted to my new laptop – a hugely expensive Apple colour PowerBook 180c. When Vivienne came in I was totally preoccupied with setting it up. She reported to Mahmoud that I was somewhat strange and was seemingly only interested in the computer! But he was proved right; Vivienne and I were married in Brighton on Friday 29th March 1996.

I absolutely loved Cambridge and recall those two years as a kaleidoscope of vivid memories, for in all kinds of ways Cambridge was a special place. Eventually I had to leave as I was on a rotation; first in Cambridge, then in Norwich and then back to Cambridge until a consultant's job became available. These don't come along very often – they're either newly created or you wait for someone to retire or die.

After those two glorious years I went to Norwich. Though it now is a teaching hospital, when I went there it was a district general hospital, which I considered a bit of a comedown after Addenbrooke's! One or two of the consultants seemed aloof and believed they were professionally superior. I soon discovered that, in fact, they were! Many of the consultants were very slick cataract surgeons and I learnt a great deal, especially from the two who had moved down from the Sunderland Eye Hospital. I also soon

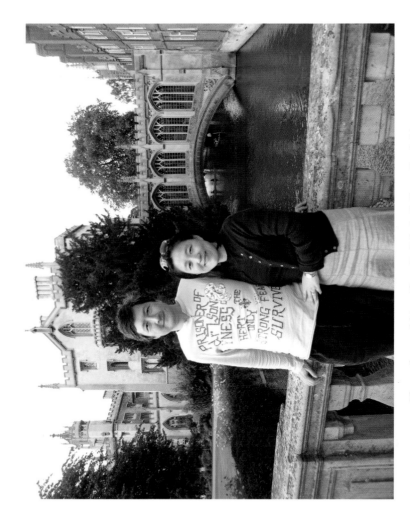

The author and his wife at St. John's College, Cambridge.

came to understand that basic science is just as important as clinical applications and techniques.

For my doctorate I focused on what can happen after a cataract is removed. The lens sits in a capsule but sometimes after surgery, residual lens cells colonise the capsule and sight fails again. With the help of my professor, George Duncan, and Michael Wormstone, his PhD student, I developed a laboratory model of the capsular bag, culturing its cells in a medium, and recorded their growth with time-lapse photography. We found we could change the medium to either encourage or suppress the growth.

Normally, if you embark on cell culture you want to grow as many cells as possible. But what we needed to do was to kill the cells, because even if a few are left they will re-colonise the capsule and obscure the implanted lens. We opened a new field and our results really made the news.

Even though I was ready to become a consultant whilst at Cambridge, I rotated to Norwich and only then applied for consultant posts. The pattern of applying has changed since then as training is shorter and much more structured. In my day it took five to six years to qualify as a doctor, followed by two to three years as a senior house officer and two to three further years as Registrar. Finally, you would be a Senior Registrar until you found a consultant post.

How many attempts would be necessary before being successful depended on how selective you were when applying. Those who wanted to stay in London almost always had a long wait, as it is a smaller catchment area and again, a post only comes up when someone has retired or died.

In 1996 everything changed. I applied to the Sussex Eye Hospital in Brighton and moved there. I found my post in

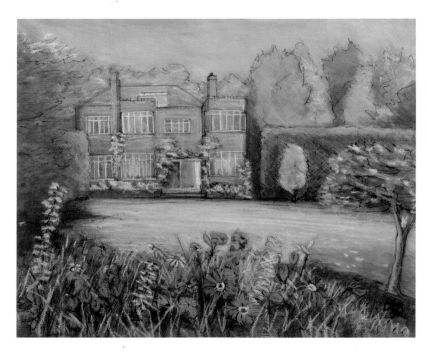

Gouache of our home and adjacent private clinic viewed from the rear garden.
Artist: Barbara Spurr.

the usual way – by reading the advertisements in the *British Medical Journal*. Really diligent people keep their ears and eyes open and find out in which hospital someone is likely to retire, or which department is going to expand. Then they make themselves known to the appropriate people and generally do a spot of self-promotion!

When applying, you send at least ten copies of your curriculum vitae and make certain the presentation is done well. Then you wait in hope of being short-listed. Generally no more than three people are interviewed. You visit and vet the place and they vet you. I remember first visiting Brighton in the summer of 1995, the weather was pleasant and so was the town. One of the things that immediately struck me about the hospital building was that it was redolent with tradition and history. I like such places, so felt I would be very comfortable there. Another reason was that I had already worked at specialist eye hospitals (Moorfields and the Western Ophthalmic) and was then – and still remain – very comfortable with that, as long as they have adequate links with the General Hospital and the Medical School, with support in both directions.

I started work at the Sussex Eye Hospital on 1st January 1996 and established my private practice four months later. Then in July 1999, Vivienne and I moved into a house in Hove, which we purchased from a former consultant (now a close friend) at the Sussex Eye Hospital. Many happy years have followed. This is also where I have set up my private clinic. As my knowledge of the eye increased so too did my wonder and amazement at its complexity.

Part III

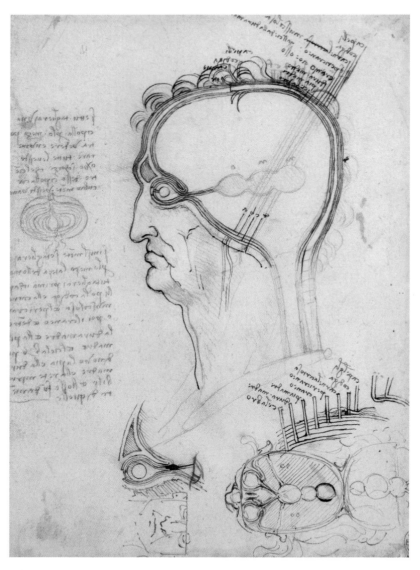

Head Section with Anatomy of the Eye Drawing, Leonardo da Vinci, Royal
Library Windsor. The Royal Collection © 2011 Her Majesty Queen Elizabeth II

74

6

The Eye

'Man is a visual animal. About half of the fibres that convey sensation to our brains stem from the optic nerves. We live in a world almost wholly orientated by sight and we seek our food, sex and shelter through information provided by our retinal images.'

The World Through Blunted Sight,
Patrick Trevor-Roper

Ten years had passed between my first job at Charing Cross and my appointment to the Sussex Eye Hospital in Brighton. Throughout all those years I was continually discovering how amazing the eye is. Exquisite in structure, unbelievably sophisticated in function and a mere 1 inch in diameter, the eye will see some 24 million different images in a lifetime – with a range of interpretation that is breathtaking.

When a child is born, the eye can focus at somewhere around the distance between the breast and a mother's face, though the resolution is poor. But soon the range will extend to infinity. We can see in bright sunlight and near darkness; we can judge speed with good accuracy and because we have two eyes, we can judge depth. The lens of each eye focuses light from the outside world on to the retina, a structure formed from a thin sheet of brain tissue that slipped into the eye during embryonic development. Each of the 130 million light sensitive retinal cells not only collects, but also analyses information about the light falling on it – a task so intensive that, gram for gram, the retina consumes six times more energy than the heart.

This alone does not give us vision, a task that falls to the main body of our brain and takes up fifty per cent of its function. Gaining a comprehensive understanding of how the brain and eye work in concert took centuries of work. Though physicians in antiquity believed that an active eye was how we saw, they had the direction of activity the wrong way round. In the fourth century BC, Plato thought that rays of light came out of the eye and seized the objects, but his student, Aristotle, was convinced that eyes received external rays of light. In the early eleventh century, Avicenna decided that the eye was merely a mirror reflecting objects in the external world.

Over the centuries more and more came to be known about the eye's anatomy, but exactly what we saw and why we saw it was never clearly understood. The first theory that involved an image being formed on the retina came in 1604 and ironically, was put forward not by a physician, nor an anatomist, but by an astronomer, Johannes Kepler. From then on there was greater emphasis on anatomy and geometry for clues about vision, and though modern cameras had not yet been invented, Kepler moved towards a camera analogy. The eye, he wrote, was a 'camera obscura' and 'vision occurs through a picture of the visible things on the white, concave surface of the retina.'

Three centuries later, the eye was likened to a pinhole

camera that produces an upside-down image. The optic
nerve transmitted the inverted image to the brain, which
then processed the information so that everything was
seen the right way up. In theories such as these the eye
was still somewhat passive – just a receiver and focuser of
light. Such models were actually too physical, paying more
attention to the effect of light on photographic plates than
they did to asking why animals need eyes and what they
need to see. One scientist suspected that if these questions
were investigated, we might understand better how the
eye actually works.

So it proved. In 1959 a scientific paper appeared which
was sensational in our understanding of sight and vision,
for it redirected our thinking and thus opened up new
fields for research. Fifty years later, 'What The Frog's Eye
Tells The Frog's Brain' is still one of the most widely cited
papers in science and its principal author, Jerome Lettvin,
of the Research Laboratory of Electronics at Massachusetts
Institute of Technology, still remains a maverick genius. By
posing the evolutionary and ecological question of what it
is important for a frog to see, Lettvin was convinced he
could reveal how the frog actually does see. The answer
was certainly not with eyes behaving like pinhole cameras.

As he pointed out, to survive a frog needs to feed. While
sitting on a lily pad, the animal is not concerned with the
stationary parts of his world, only moving parts, such as
flies. Compared to the complex human eye that is constantly moving and always monitoring the external world,
a frog's eye is not so complex and the retina's connections
to the brain far simpler. Whereas earlier scientists tried to
find out how the frog's eye worked by subjecting it to
flashing lights or electrical currents, Jerome Lettvin argued
that one should show it small moving objects.

In evolutionary terms this makes great sense. A frog ignores all stationary objects around it. Even food like insects or worms will only be captured provided they move, and indeed Lettvin and his colleagues found that a frog could be fooled by anything moving – even an inedible pinhead.

Lettvin's new question generated new experiments, which generated new results and a major discovery. The retina was far from being a mere receptor of light and a transmitter of images; an enormous amount of sophisticated discrimination was actually taking place there, way before any impulses reached the brain. Rather than merely transmitting a more or less accurate copy of the distribution of light as it hits the eye's receptor cells, the retina 'speaks to the brain in a language already highly organised and interpreted'. The frog's eye is actually telling the frog's brain about its external world, and so too does the highly complex, exquisite structure that is the human eye.

There are two types of light-sensitive retinal cells known as rods and cones. They have been described as nature's microchips; millions of them constantly transmit electrochemical messages along fibre optic strands in the nerves. The cones handle fine details and colour and spring to attention the instant the light hits them. The rods are the laggards. When we enter a dim or darkened room, they take several minutes to come to maximum sensitivity and besides helping us see in the dark, they allow us to distinguish between black and white. The rods and the cones are connected by bipolar cells, whose job is to relay the messages to over one million ganglion cells which transmit messages to the brain, where they are finally decoded.

The system is in a continuous frenzy of activity. Thirty different areas in the brain act in concert to analyse the various features of the data sent from our eyes. One area puts names to faces; another processes the 10 million colours we see – and so on for every feature we can discern. Literally in the blink of an eye the brain is able to synthesise the three dimensional world out there, a world that we not only observe in vivid colour and high resolution, but one we understand, in which we can navigate, whose beauty we can appreciate and even reproduce in painting.

The scale of the task and the discrimination required is huge. A policeman has spotted a likely suspect in the sunlight. But then the suspect dives into a subway and in its dim light, the blue of his jacket is no longer the same blue as it was in daylight. The colour of his hair has changed, and so too has his shadow on the ground. In terms of visual properties he is entirely transformed. If the man turns his face to one side, the features that the officer committed to memory are now distorted, so he must map a new set of facial features in order to obtain a match. Yet still he can track him.

At the rate of millions of calculations a second, the brain can identify where the image of the suspect ends and the background begins. Once the boundaries have been determined, the officer can gauge how fast this man-shaped collection of pinpricks of data is moving, how far away he is and what direction he is planning to take.

Such calculations are conducted every second of our waking life. We know nothing of this activity nor are we overwhelmed by the huge amount of information. All this testifies to the remarkable ability of the human brain to process – not singly but simultaneously – a myriad of features in the world around us.

Depth, colour, motion, edge detection, identity – all give

form and structure to what we are seeing. But we have to make sense of it all. Who, or what, are we looking at? Here is where our past experience comes in. Based on what we have seen before, we recognise, identify and classify what we are seeing now. From birth we accumulate experience and this defines both us and our world and what we make of it. The eyes most certainly have it. Of course, sometimes things go wrong.

* * *

Though naturally I am happy to treat any eye problem, I am really most comfortable dealing with the front of the eye. This is somewhat ironic because I was attracted into the field because of my short sight and thought the front of the eye a very minor region. How wrong I was.

So what is its precise structure? Every single part of the eye has a function and a purpose. The eyebrows afford protection. If you are knocked on the face, they take the brunt of the blow even though the lower part of the eye can also take some injury. The brow is also there to deflect rain.

The eyelids blink and blinking keeps the surface of the eye moist. This is essential, for if the eye dries, it shrivels. So while the eyelids don't look like windscreen wipers, the function is not dissimilar.

Next is the cornea, the clear part of the eye that covers the coloured regions. It is similar to a watch glass and provides a clear window. Being very convex the cornea is optically active and bends the light to a focus at the back of the eye.

The cornea and the white of the eye merge at the limbus, where the corneal stem cells live. If this area is badly damaged, then the layer of healthy cells replenishing the surface of the cornea can be lost.

THE EYE

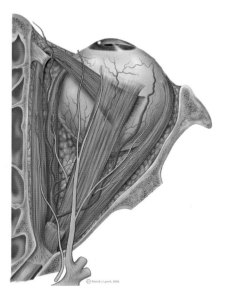

Anatomy of the orbit as viewed from above showing the eye, extraocular muscles, orbital blood vessels (red) and nerves (yellow).

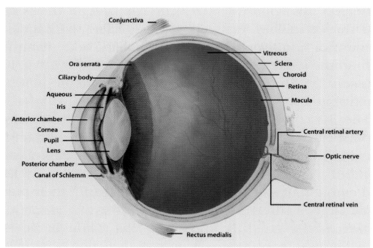

Cross sectional diagram showing the internal anatomy of the eye.
Both diagrams courtesy of Wikimedia.

In fact the cornea has three main layers. At the front, the epithelium that faces the outside world is one of several areas where cells do replenish themselves. Provided the damage is minor, a scratch on the epithelium will heal quickly. The next layer, the stroma, forms the main body of the cornea. Yet though it can remodel itself, it cannot replenish. Finally, the endothelium is a layer at the back that acts like a pump and pushes water out of the stroma to keep everything clear. It, too, cannot replenish itself, so if the back layer of the cornea is damaged by disease, trauma or even bad cataract surgery, it becomes swollen and the sight blurs. Even if the cornea is merely waterlogged, the overlying epithelial cells become loose and detach, the nerve endings are irritated and the eye becomes painful. So this complex, beautiful, three-layered window, which is only half a millimetre in thickness, is absolutely vital for sight.

Behind this window – between the back of the cornea and the crystalline lens – is a space filled with aqueous humour, a liquid produced by the ciliary body lying just behind the lens. If this becomes diseased the eye will lose pressure, will not keep its shape, will become soft and squidgy and the optics will go awry.

The iris – the coloured part of the eye – is actually a sophisticated muscle. When its circular fibres contract the pupil becomes smaller, when the radial fibres contract the pupil dilates and both movements are controlled by light and emotion. If someone becomes very fearful their pupils grow large, as they do when you feel a strong attraction.

Next is the crucially important lens. Though the lens actually gives proportionally less optical power than the cornea, the critical fact is that its optical power can change with accommodation. A contraction of the ciliary body muscle triggers changes in the shape of the lens and this allows us to focus from distance to near and very quickly back to distance again.

Other mechanisms trigger the changing shape of the lens. If you look at something in the distance, the eyes no longer converge. They are further apart, in parallel with each other while viewing, so the eye muscles and the brain know you are looking further away. Both then make adjustments.

As we look from distance to close up, three things happen. First, the eyes converge; second, the lens bulges and becomes thicker, and so its focus changes; finally the pupils become smaller. This three-part mechanism is called the oculomotor triad and is served by the third cranial nerve that emerges from the brain and ends behind the eye.

Behind the lens is the vitreous cavity, a gelatinous body that actually does very little. However, it can be a problem in old age or with short sightedness when it can degenerate and liquefy. Sometimes it even peels away from the retina and optical impurities, seen as floaters, then appear in the jelly. When this happens it can even tear the retina and cause it to become detached.

Finally, at the very back of the eye is the retina itself, which acts like a photographic film, though the analogy is by no means perfect. Every signal from the retina – whether electrical or chemical – goes through the photoreceptors and bipolar cells and all eventually pour into a bunch of cables formed from smaller nerve fibres. These, one million of them, join to form the optic nerve that connects to the brain. At some point near the pituitary gland, half the fibres cross over or *decussate*, which means that your left brain serves your right visual environment and vice versa.

Behind the retina lies the choroid, a network of blood vessels that sometimes grow forward and break through a membrane under the retina causing macular degeneration, a medical condition that usually affects older adults because of damage to the retina. Macular degeneration can make it difficult or impossible to read or recognise faces, although enough peripheral vision remains to allow other activities of daily life.

Behind the choroid is the sclera, the white of the eye, part of which you see when you look at an eye directly.

All this is contained in an organ just under an inch or 2.5 cm in diameter, though when operating using binocular microscopes this can seem surprisingly big. Yet the volume of the anterior chamber, which is bounded by the back of the cornea and iris, is only one quarter of a cubic centimetre and a cataract surgeon has to work within that space. Moreover, it is absolutely vital not to break the very thin posterior capsule, which is only a few microns in thickness.

These are just some of the levels at which we work. However, we can go even further into the structures already mentioned. A deeper look with an electron microscope, followed by a study of the biochemistry, reveals a higher degree of exquisite complexity. I don't pretend to know it all; no one does. But I do know that the constraints on effective cataract surgery include not only the anatomy of the structures, and being able to see them in magnification, but also being able to appreciate their spatial dimensions.

There are a multitude of reasons why I have found my profession absolutely fascinating, even though I deal with one of the most common problems of the eye – cataract.

7

The Changing World of Cataract Surgery

Cataract surgery is the most common surgery in the world. In Western societies, cataracts – the increasing thickness and cloudiness of the lens – are mainly caused by three factors; age, gender (being more frequent in females) and diabetes. But globally there are other factors that come into play, such as episodes of acute dehydration or exposure to intense ultraviolet light, radiation, or trauma, perhaps from a punch during a fight. In addition, steroid tablets taken for the treatment of asthma or arthritis can provoke cataracts. There are also genetic conditions, some babies are even born with cataracts.

As we pointed out earlier, cataract surgery has been performed for generations. The first extremely primitive technique was 'couching', where the surgeon waited for the cataract to ripen and then it was 'pushed' so hard that it was – hopefully – dislocated into the vitreous humour. Surgeons started wearing surgical loupes, which allowed a magnified view of the cataract, ensuring a more complete removal. Whatever the method used, the patient had to wear thick glasses to see anything at all.

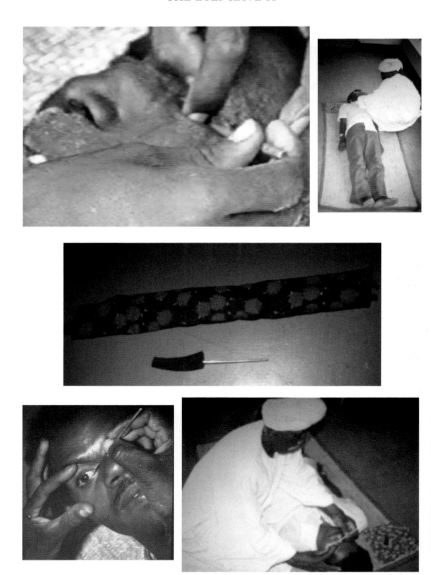

Couching of cataract as practised in Sudan recently. Courtesy of Mr Nick Astbury, PRCOphth, and Dr A. Basha.

Eventually three inventions changed everything. The first was the binocular operating microscope that allowed the surgeon to see with both eyes. It made its first appearance in eye surgery in the early 1950s when Professor H. Harms of the eye clinic in Tubingen, Germany, working with the Carl Zeiss Company, became the first person to publish his experiences with the machine. In Britain, early exponents of this new tool were Dermot Pierse working in Croydon and Michael Roper-Hall working in Birmingham. By the 1960s the instrument became more accepted and after 1975 was in common use.

As the surgeon was now using both eyes, he could not only see the structures magnified but could also judge depth in fine, three-dimensional detail. There have been no major advances in the operating microscope since then, but there have been several important refinements. These include improved optics, coaxial lighting (illumination in the line of the surgeon's sight), motorised focusing and magnification, extra eyepiece for assistant surgeon, and video camera attachment so others such as the scrub nurse can follow the procedure.

The second significant invention was monofilament nylon stitches, actually thinner than human hair. The wonderful thing about nylon is that unlike silk, which was used earlier, the sutures are quite elastic and don't create inflammation. (This is one reason why patients can start moving around much sooner, and don't have to lie immobile in bed to avoid disturbance to the wound.) These nylon stitches are pre-mounted on a curved needle looking like a hook. There's no eye, because the nylon is already inside the metal. Since the needle is curved you bring it through the tissue in a circular motion.

All these remarkable changes, whether style of surgery

or delicate instrumentation, have had a direct impact on healing. Years ago, patients would have to remain in bed in a dark room for two weeks following cataract surgery, with their head completely immobilised so the wound was not disturbed. The operation was quite bloody and much trauma to the surrounding blood vessels was created, so the sutures were heavy. The success rate was low and often complications followed. When the eye had finally settled down the patient would be fitted with very thick post-cataract spectacles made of heavy glass, just like the bottom of a jam jar (or contact lenses since the 1930s). Such thick glasses caused much distortion of distance and proportion, so people could miss a step in a flight of stairs, or grasp for a door handle that was five inches to the left or right of where they had placed their hand. It was certainly not the best rehabilitation of vision. Nowadays, they can go home and move around almost immediately.

Today we are able to do far more complicated surgery with smaller and smaller wounds, so healing is much more rapid and disturbance to the function and shape – and therefore the optics – of the eye is significantly reduced. Moreover, since the wounds are both very small and self-sealing, thus requiring no suturing, they are much less likely to burst if any trauma should occur later. Recently, I did a successful emergency operation on a lady who had fallen and ruptured her eyeball right along the large wound of the old-style cataract operation. Had she fallen after modern surgery, the wound would not have ruptured in the first place.

But the third, really significant change was the introduction of plastic artificial lenses – a huge improvement on spectacles made of thick glass. This development was initiated by Sir Harold Ridley, an ophthalmic surgeon at St

Thomas' Hospital, in association with Rayner's, an established optical firm in Brighton and Hove. Rayner celebrated its centenary in 2010 and still makes enormous contributions to ophthalmology. Their primary product is intraocular lenses used in cataract and related ophthalmic surgery.

Today the company consists of two very different elements. One is retail; it owns some 140 opticians' shops, mostly trading under the name Rayner. Historically this is the main part of their business; the firm began in 1910 as a high street optician in Vere Street, just off Cavendish Square, London, started by Mr Reiner and Mr Keeler. Reiner's father was from Germany, but during World War One the directors anglicised the company name to Rayner & Keeler Ltd . In 1917, Mr Keeler left and started a separate company that still exists today.

In order to keep the business growing, they encouraged eye surgeons to come to the shop to fit their patients with spectacles. So Rayner's began to make trial sets of glasses – small frames with a slot in them – as well as other optical devices such as ophthalmoscopes, so surgeons could look directly into the eye. These were not made in Vere Street but in a workshop in Kemp Town, Brighton. Mr Reiner eventually moved to Brighton where he became a Town Councillor.

During World War One, their workshop was requisitioned and all activities were directed towards the war effort. Amongst other devices, the company made trench periscopes and also diversified into 'gemmology' – optical devices for examining the qualities of sapphires, rubies etc. By the 1920s Rayner's was a very successful business that was soon working closely with the Sussex Eye Hospital.

Harold Ridley, the son of a surgeon, was educated at Cambridge and held consultant positions at both St Thomas' Hospital and Moorfields. By the 1930s he was

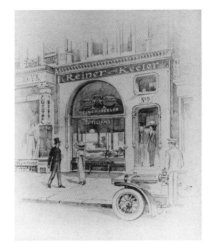

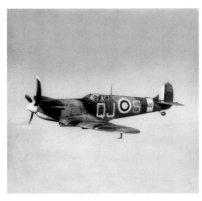

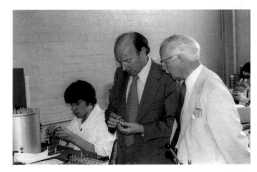

Top left: Reiner shop front.

Top right: Spitfire aircraft.

Middle: Harold Ridley (right) and John Ingham.

Bottom: Sir Harold Ridley knighted by Her Majesty the Queen.

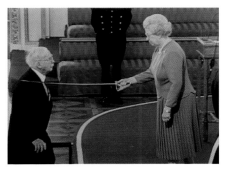

Images courtesy of Rayner Intraocular Lenses Limited.

considered a most eminent, though unassuming, young consultant who would go on to make a major contribution to cataract surgery. However, he was very modest and always gave credit to a young student, Steve Parry. One day, Parry was watching the removal of a cataract for the very first time. After the operation was over, the young man said to Ridley, 'What a pity you cannot fit a plastic or artificial lens in its place.'

During World War Two, Ridley treated many fighter pilots at Moorfields during the Battle of Britain. There is one well-documented case of a pilot, Flight Lieutenant 'Mouse' Cleaver, who had baled out over Winchester and was blinded in one eye, with serious injuries in the other. This had been his second sortie that day; he wasn't in his own plane – he had been scrambled quickly and told to run to another Hurricane as his engine wouldn't start. He was flying without eye protection.

Enemy gunfire passed through the canopy of the Hurricane and some fragments of Perspex windscreen had entered his eyes. What Ridley would observe was that if fragments had entered the eye there would indeed be damage, but in one sense they were tolerated as this plastic is a biocompatible substance and causes no inflammation.

Ridley was certainly a very clever man. Many of his contemporaries believed that it was his logic that connected an injury in an eye with the possibility of making an artificial lens of neutral plastic. But he would always insist, 'No, it wasn't my idea: it was this young student Steve Parry who asked why I didn't implant an artificial lens.'

The use of an artificial lens was not an entirely new idea. In 1795 the court oculist in Dresden, called Casa Amata, had experimented by replacing a cataract with a glass implant. Nevertheless, using the same kind of plastic as in the canopies of Hurricanes really was new and it was certainly Ridley's idea. During 1948, Ridley was frequently at Rayner's talking with John Pike, the company's optical director.

Ridley suggested that the firm discussed the problem with the people who made Perspex. Fortunately, not only did John Pike know this was ICI, but he had an influential contact there, Dr John Holt. As a result, ICI agreed to make a small, high quality run of essentially the same plastic as used in aeroplanes. In 1952, one of their very early lenses was implanted in a young girl, aged twelve, who had been hit by a ball while playing. Her surgeon in Johannesburg, Dr Edward 'Teddy' Epstein, was a disciple of Harold Ridley's. Today, sixty years later, the patient is around seventy and still has the original implant in her eye. The lens is absolutely clear and not discoloured in any way. She sees very well; her retina is not damaged either by sunlight or ultraviolet radiation. There is no other material presently used in implants – whether for hips or dental work – that has such a successful reputation for longevity. It does what it is intended to do from day one. Ridley lived to a ripe old age and was knighted in the Millennium Honours List. He died the following year, aged 94.

People often ask if a cataract will grow back – it will not. During surgery the posterior capsule is left in place to support the new lens implant. Sometimes cells colonise the posterior capsule and while the patient sees clearly for quite a while, eventually the cells grow in multiple layers, deposit protein and light starts to scatter again. The treatment is to destroy the cells growing back with a laser beam, thus creating an opening so the eye can see again.

The need for this procedure is much more frequent in children because they (and their cells) are growing very actively! Unlike for adults, a general anaesthetic is necessary when operating as they would find it very difficult to remain still throughout the procedure.

Many things come into play before new machines in medicine become popular and widespread. Before they can be licensed for medical use, large costs have to be met, covering development and safety requirements. Manufacturers want to see a return on their investment. Yet while new technology places a burden on health resources, the therapeutic advantages are often significant.

There have been significant innovations in other areas as well, all vital for the surgeon and worlds away from needling out a solid cataract with a lancet. First there are the instruments and machinery. During cataract surgery you are using not only your hands but your feet too, on separate pieces of machinery. While the right and left hands are manipulating instruments, the left foot is operating a pedal that allows you to move the microscope in various directions or to focus, to increase or decrease the magnification or the lighting level. Sometimes you are resting on your heel, sometimes on the ball of the foot. On the right pedal there is an accelerator with three positions: on position zero, nothing happens; on position one, irrigating fluid is going into the eye, keeping the eye inflated, dissipating heat created by ultrasound, and flushing away unwanted debris; on position two, you could be activating the ultrasound vibration which fragments the cataract, or aspirating fluid and debris out of the eye, depending on the mode of the machine, and so on. Once you are in position two, the harder you press, the more ultrasound energy is released, or the more suction is created, much like a car's accelerator pedal. You can also move your right foot sideways to set the machine into many different functions.

A novice cataract surgeon has a lot to learn just to master the coordination of their hands and their feet!

The machine that enables us to do this has to be built in such a way that though you are resting on your behind, you can move all four limbs freely. Armrests on some operating chairs provide a means to rest your elbows. Positioning your little fingers on part of the patient's forehead means you are moving with them, should they inadvertently shift their head.

It is not only surgical competence, dexterity and understanding that are important, but also positioning. Eye surgeons often suffer from neck and back problems. It is important to relax and stop any muscular spasms forming.

There have been many more innovations in the way that cataract surgery is delivered and, once again, differences from the past are marked. 'Cataract surgery by appointment' is an extreme but well-liked form of day case surgery. Before a patient arrives for their cataract surgery, they can put in the pupil-dilating eye drops themselves and, unlike other operations, do not have to fast beforehand. They are asked to arrive with a clean face, wearing no make-up or nail varnish; they are led straight into the operating theatre at the appointed time, stay in their own clothes, and are in and out within half an hour; they don't need to go through a pre-op ward and relatives can watch the operation on a TV screen in an adjacent coffee room. If the relatives are a little squeamish they can avert their eyes from one television screen and watch something else on another. So it's rather like being in a restaurant where the chef is happy to let you see what is going on in the kitchen! Everyone feels more confident because there's nothing to hide.

Setting schedules in this way can of course cause problems. You ask people to come in at a specific time but if the surgeon is encountering problems and takes much longer on one operation, the whole programme is temporarily disrupted. Sometimes you are delayed because someone else is occupying the theatre; sometimes the patient arrives late, or not at all, and the whole surgical team has to wait around for the next patient to turn up. I am happy to say that this is rare; since we developed 'Cataract Surgery by Appointment' in 2002 I have only had one no-show.

There is one final innovation that I support wholeheartedly and that is doing both eyes at the same time, in a procedure we call 'immediately sequential bilateral cataract surgery'. I advocate it, although there is much resistance in the field.

The advantages are numerous; one pre-assessment, one visit to the operating theatre, just one period to reach stability before the patient can get new glasses, the time that carers have to commit is reduced, it is cheaper because there is less moving about, theatre time is decreased as the patient is already in place and so you just move from one eye to the next. To sum up, it's very good for the patient, carers, society and health economics.

An objection that is constantly raised is that both eyes, not just one, will be placed at surgical risk. We never try to persuade patients who are reluctant to have both eyes done together, and we make the procedures thoroughly safe. First of all, only routine (i.e. not complex) cases of cataract surgery are offered this option. Second, we make it quite clear that it's not like firing a missile. We do not press a button and hey presto, both eyes have been done at the same time. On the contrary; if the first eye has not gone well we don't proceed with the second, but stop and reconsider. We see how the patient feels and how the first eye is behaving, then we re-schedule. So whereas the procedure used to be called 'simultaneous bilateral' surgery, we insist that it is not simultaneous; it is 'immediately sequential' – this means there is a choice whether or not to proceed.

Thirdly, to prevent cross-infection, indeed any infection at all, nothing at all is used on both eyes. So after finishing the first eye, we re-scrub, change our gloves and gowns, move to a new trolley of instruments which has gone through a completely different sterilisation cycle and been held back from the previous week. All the solutions, chemicals and other things that go inside the eye will have come from different manufacturers, or will have different batch numbers.

No surgical procedure is completely safe. But for people who want it, doing both eyes together should be an option. Perhaps those who disagree are basing their response both on a gut feeling and on advice given during their training to wait a while before doing the second eye. The evidence tells us that the risk of both eyes going blind is only one in 200,000. Another safety factor is that we re-assess after the first eye is done and if we have *any* hesitation, we do not proceed with the second eye. We have an incredibly safe protocol. Other eye operations involve doing both eyes at the same time; squint, retinal detachment and laser refractive surgery are examples.

A final issue arises with private patients' insurance companies. They regard both eyes done in one sitting as one-and-a-half operations rather than two, so give a correspondingly reduced cover. In fact the stress and elaborate preparations for the surgical team mean that their work is in no way reduced and failure to provide cover is not acceptable to hospital and surgeon alike.

Immediately sequential bilateral cataract surgery is something I will continue to work on because I believe it is a really effective way of delivering treatment and is likely to become increasingly popular.

* * *

My desire to become an eye surgeon came about indirectly through my painting. Throughout my career I have never lost my interest in art. As I studied cataracts, a fascinating connection appeared that provided an absorbing contrast to the daily round of technical detail and surgical procedures. My interest in this has remained constant, as over the years I have collected a number of paintings.

I especially like Impressionist and post-Impressionist paintings. These artists are particularly fascinating since some have argued that their styles originated in eye problems that developed gradually throughout their lives. As he became older, Monet began to paint the Japanese bridge in his garden more abstractly, increasingly blurred and dark. I am a Francophile and we have a hideaway in Normandy, an area frequented by many of these artists, so we often visit Monet's home and gardens. It is also fortunate that we live in Brighton, because neighbouring Rottingdean was previously an enclave of artists, as well as poets and writers.

Patrick Trevor-Roper, a distinguished ophthalmologist, wrote a classic work on art and defective vision, *The World Through Blunted Sight*. Some of his conclusions are controversial; some people do not accept the connections he makes, nor the conclusions he draws. Nevertheless, his questions and ideas are challenging. For example, in the chapter 'The Withdrawal of Colours' he devotes a whole section to the effects of acquired colour blindness that can

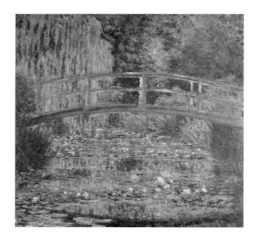

Monet's painting of the Japanese bridge at the gardens of his home in Giverny, France.

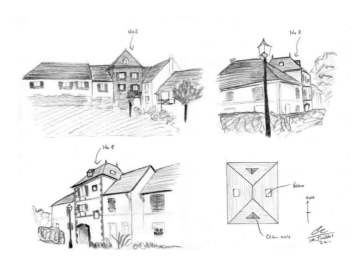

The author's sketches of his hideaway in Normandy.

develop through a number of eye disorders. This is especially true of cataracts, when the increasing opacity in the lens has the effect of imposing a colour filter between the retina and the outside world. The colours that are filtered out vary from patient to patient, but as the cataract advances the shorter wavelengths of light – violet and blue – become absorbed and eventually only red rays reach the retina. Once the cataract has been removed and a new lens fitted, patients often record an immediate increase in their blue vision.

A few days after an artist patient received cataract surgery, he twice painted a vase of flowers that was beside his bed, once with each eye. The contrast between the reddish colours from his un-operated eye and the bluish colours seen with the operated eye was overwhelming. Another artist went through a pink period and his concentration on this colour was entirely due to his cataracts. His paintings fetched really high prices, but after the operation his pink period ended and the prices dropped significantly.

Monet developed cataract, and Trevor-Roper claims that the resultant changes in his vision are obvious in his series of final paintings. His whites and blues began pure and realistic, but gradually the whites and even the greens became yellowish, while the blues moved towards purple. Monet was in despair and wrote, 'Reds appeared muddy to me, pinks insipid, and the intermediate or lower tones escaped me. What I painted was more and more dark, more like an "old picture" ... and when I compared it to my former works, I would be seized by a frantic rage and slash all my canvases with a penknife.'

His final pictures, including *The Water Garden at Giverny*, were done after 1920 by which time he was eighty years old and his sight was beginning to fail. In 1923, George Clemençeau, who had twice been Prime Minister of France, persuaded Monet to have cataract surgery and he agreed, even though he was aware that the operations on two other artists, Daumier and Mary Cassatt, had been unsuccessful. Once home, Monet had the familiar sensation of diffuse blueness and was surprised at 'the strange colours' of his most recent pictures. He felt that up to that point he had been painting 'through an opaque glass', as indeed he had. His new powerful lens gave him limited sight, but there was also distortion of both shape and colour. Nevertheless the outcome was reasonably satisfactory, because he returned to painting with great enthusiasm. However, his landscapes became violent, increasingly febrile and hallucinated, with red and blue unnaturally predominant. When finally Monet was no longer able to see yellow, he gave up his art altogether, saying, 'the painter having been operated on for cataract must renounce painting.' Fortunately, with our modern techniques such self-sacrifice is no longer necessary. I have many artist patients who have returned to painting following successful cataract surgery.

Some patients painted the lovely experiences they had while actually having cataract surgery and these have been published. After the local anaesthetic that blunts the optic nerve, artists under cataract surgery see beautiful swirly coloured patterns when the bright light comes on, although the eye soon settles down.

It is not only after eye operations that the artist's view of the world can change. Others with multiple sclerosis or neuritis have painted how their world appears. Initially everything breaks up into dots, almost like an Impressionist painting, but as they recover, the world they

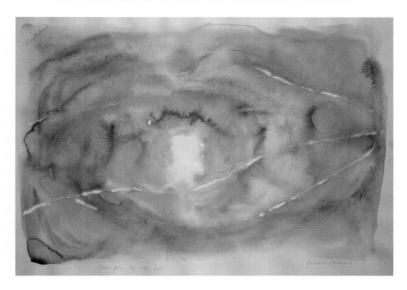

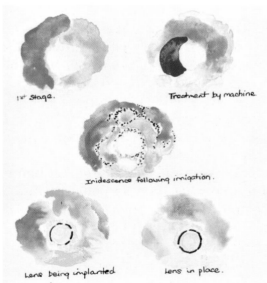

Visual experience during cataract surgery under topical anaesthesia. Courtesy of the *British Medical Journal*.

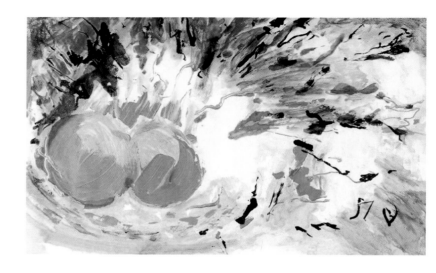

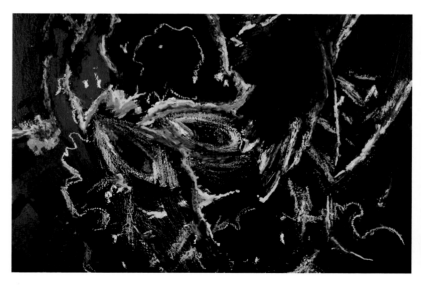

Visual perception during cataract surgery under local anaesthesia. Courtesy of the *British Journal of Ophthalmology*.

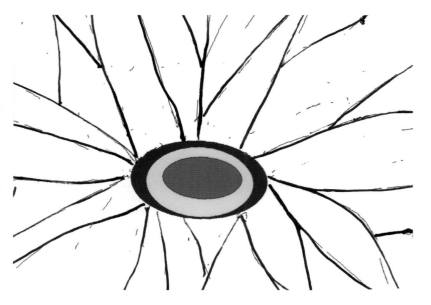

The author's patient, Gill Pettifor, an artist, captures what she saw during her cataract operation. 'The white shards emanating from the intense colour were very white and shimmery – difficult to represent.'

perceive soon seems smoother and more realistic. When the brain malfunctions, patients can experience double and triple vision, or a doubling or tripling of images, even see things that are not there at all.

I remain fascinated by all of this, indeed with all of art. I have so many questions but my fundamental one is this; why don't artists paint the world exactly as it really is? I am sure we do paint as we see, but why should any altered or defective sight not have the same effect on the canvas as it does on the real world? I think this may be a technical issue. We paint something that actually has altered, but to us appears the same as what we see.

8

Life at the Cutting Edge

Whether it is the millions of people who suffer from cataract or the very few who go blind from rare conditions, whether genetic or a result of trauma, the consequent devastation and loss of quality of life is the same. At one end of the scale we do over 3000 cataract operations a year at the Sussex Eye Hospital. At the other end, since we are the national referral centre for osteo-odonto-keratoprosthesis surgery (OOKP), we undertake one particular, highly specialised and difficult operation about six times a year. We are the only hospital in Britain to offer the procedure and since the surgery is so complicated and infrequently required, it makes huge sense for the practices and expertise to be concentrated in one centre of excellence.

This OOKP is offered to people who cannot take corneal transplants so, before describing it, we should examine what these transplants are. Suitable patients include those who have corneal distortion, or clouding because of immune disease, infection or trauma. Transplantation is then a viable option and everyone is aware of the consequent problems, which essentially boil down to rejection. It used to be said that since a healthy cornea has no blood vessels it has immune privilege, that is to say it is out of reach of the immune system and can therefore avoid being rejected. But that's not strictly true, for the cells of the immune system are not totally dependent upon the blood vessels to take them round the body. They can travel through the aqueous humour, land on the back of the cornea and start rejecting any donated material.

The rejection process can happen at any time and only seventy per cent of corneal transplantations survive for five years. We always urge people who have had a corneal transplant to seek attention the moment there is any sign of rejection – such as the eye reddening, the sight blurring, or discomfort and sensitivity to light. If caught early, rejection can be treated with hourly steroid eye drops.

We are always very selective about the patient's suitability. If a person has one good eye and the other has corneal blindness that could be cured with a transplant, the trend is just to leave well alone since intervention could bring new problems. Complications from corneal transplantation range from infection, wound instability and astigmatism to immune rejections.

If a transplant operation is advisable, we normally use a punch to take out a circular disc from the central part of the cornea. Then we punch a slightly larger disc from the donated cornea and stitch it in with nylon sutures. Nowadays we can be very selective and actually decide which layers of the cornea to transplant. For example, if the endothelium is healthy but there is a scar in the stroma, we simply replace that part. However, if the endothelium is depleted we can put in a new donor endothelium on a thin carrier of stroma.

We can also transplant corneal (limbal) epithelial stem cells. If one eye only has been injured with say a chemical burn and the surface cells fail to heal because of a deficiency of limbal stem cells, it is possible to harvest stem cells from the other, healthy eye for transplantation. Without exception, one has to be extremely careful. Sometimes an eye can look sound but still be damaged and if you then remove stem cells from that, then the patient might end up with two poor eyes.

Nowadays it is possible to take a much smaller sample of reserve stem cells from the good eye, grow them in laboratory culture and then transplant them. In this process – called *ex-vivo* expansion – you are actually taking a mixture of stem cells and transient amplifying cells, the daughter cells of stem cells. The cells grow in laboratory culture and spread across a circular disc on a carrier, such as an amniotic or man-made membrane. Then the disc is separated from its carrier and popped onto the recipient eye, almost like a contact lens, and it will take. This procedure entails a far smaller risk to the donor eye. Where both eyes have stem cell deficiency, the same process can be applied to stem cells obtained from a donor.

There is considerable and constant demand for donated corneas. In one respect, eye donation is unique. A donated kidney or heart must be fresh when taken and in both cases the surgeon must move fast. However, eyes, or just the cornea, can be taken up to twelve hours following death, so the relatives of the donor need have no worries about anything being removed before the person is dead. If, as sometimes happens, the deceased has indicated that they want to be a multi-organ donor, the cornea is harvested last of all.

Though there is a consistent call for donors, not everyone can become one. Some people are ruled out by having blood-borne infections such as hepatitis, HIV or neurological diseases. Eyes that have had surgery or been traumatised are also unsuitable. Nevertheless, donated organs can still be used for research and teaching. When someone elects to donate their eyes there are three separate consent boxes; therapeutic use, teaching and research. Normally we hope all three will be ticked.

When successful, the consequences of corneal transplants are wonderful. For example, Fuchs' corneal dystrophy is a progressive disease that makes the cornea swell in both eyes. Vision becomes blurred and if left untreated, great pain and blindness follows. In this condition corneal transplantation can be hugely successful.

However, if the patient's eyes are too damaged for a corneal transplant to survive, then there is only one alternative – for which the Sussex Eye Hospital is the only centre in Britain – an operation involving the creation of an artificial cornea.

Anyone told that someone's sight might be restored by the use of one of his or her teeth would be totally incredulous. Such a procedure was invented almost fifty years ago in Rome where I first learned the technique, though it has been gradually modified over the years. OOKP is a two-stage operation, and since each stage takes about six hours each one is done quite separately. The procedure involves harvesting a tooth, its root and surrounding bone and shaping them into a window frame into which a Perspex optical cylinder is sited, through which the patient sees.

The crux of the operation involves deceit; fooling the immune system into believing that the small, Perspex cylinder which forms part of the artificial cornea is not a foreign body. The cylinder is embedded into the tooth and it is the tooth that does the fooling, the only part of the body that can!

I learnt the procedure from Professor Giancarlo Falcinelli, my Italian ophthalmology teacher. Now in his eighties, he and his son, also an ophthalmologist, travelled the world to get people started in this surgery. The first time I heard about them was in 1993 at a meeting in Bordeaux, when I saw different techniques for tackling the basic problem of treating blindness in people who cannot take corneal transplants.

Of the dozen or so techniques available, I selected OOKP because it gave better results, both in terms of retention and long-term vision. I met Falcinelli again in December 1993 at a meeting that combined a series of serious surgical lectures in Italian and English and was strangely, but not unpleasantly, interspersed with parties and opera.

In 1994 I went to Rome again for four weeks. Having absorbed fifty-two hours of language tuition I was not fluent, but nevertheless equipped to tackle the challenge. I had a list of questions; I interviewed Falcinelli's OOKP patients and was able to examine them, which confirmed excellent long-term surgical results. The whole experience was wonderful. After I was appointed at Brighton I explained that OOKP was one of the procedures I was keen to perform and over time, did more and more of the operations.

The first stage of surgery involves removing superficial scar tissue from the cornea of the blind eye, and covering the whole eye surface with a flap of skin taken from inside the cheek.

Then a canine – generally the tooth of choice for this procedure – is removed from the jaw, along with its root and a small block of jawbone. If a patient does not have their own teeth they can ask a relative for a tooth donation,

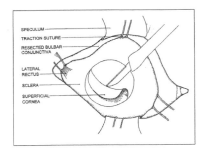
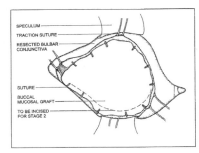

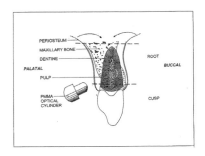
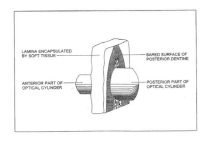

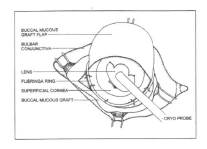
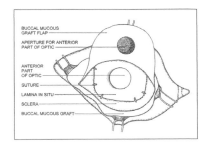

Line drawings depicting the steps of OOKP surgery.
Reproduced from *Eye News*.

or a piece of bone can be taken from somewhere else. Neither of these are as good as the patient's own tooth. The tooth root and its surrounding bone are then shaped into a rectangular plate into which a Perspex optical cylinder (which acts as a lens) is cemented. This is placed under the muscle beneath the lower eyelid of the other eye, where it remains for two to four months, during which time tissue grows around the whole construction.

This may seem a long time, and inconvenient too, but those undergoing this operation have great patience, because although they have lost their sight they now have the prospect of regaining it. Finally the previously transplanted flap of inside cheek skin over the blind eye is raised and a hole is made through both its centre and that of the cornea. The holes allow both ends of the optical cylinder to poke through, allowing the patient to see. Then the plate containing the tooth and the optical cylinder, which now has a healthy growth of tissue around it, is inserted into the hole with the cylinder protruding slightly. The process is hugely challenging. Between two-thirds and three-quarters of the operations are successful, but sometimes the retina or optic nerves fail to function properly.

The operation was filmed for BBC TV's *Tomorrow's World* in 1996/7 and Professor Falcinelli came over for the occasion. Indeed, he did almost the whole procedure though I was handed certain stages.

I have done this now about sixty times, supported by a dedicated team, including my dear maxillo-facial surgical colleague Jim Herold. One of my most successful patients is a forty-two year old man, a former builder from Rotherham in South Yorkshire, who had been blind for twelve years after a tub of aluminium exploded in his face. His left eye had to be removed and he was told that he

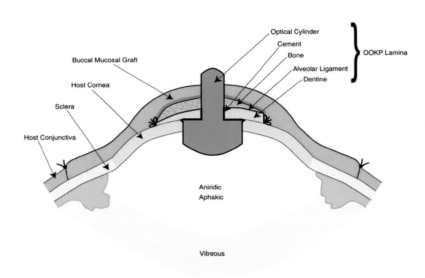

Cross section anatomy of the OOKP eye.

would never see with his right eye either. He met his wife when already blind. Afterwards he said, 'The first person I wanted to see was my wife. The doctors took the bandages off and it was like looking through water... and then I saw this figure and it was her. It was unbelievable.'

We have disseminated the technique worldwide. I have demonstrated it in Japan, India and Singapore and intend to do so in Poland and America.

* * *

Today, there is a great deal of research at the very cutting edge of science into ways to help blind people. The advent of lasers was a major innovation making many new surgical techniques possible and providing a huge contribution to the advance of many ophthalmological procedures.

Lasers can cut, melt, blast and explode – all very precisely. There are actually many types and though all work differently, they have many common characteristics for their waves form a very narrow, focused (coherent) beam whose peaks and troughs are all coordinated. Where white light consists of a spectrum of seven traditional colours, lasers are all of pure colour.

Lasers for diabetic retinopathy

The xenon arc was one of the very first lasers, in fact not so much a laser as a very strong light. This was the forerunner of thermal lasers used for the treatment of diabetic retinopathy, a condition when the blood vessels are insufficient to supply the oxygen the retina demands. As the retina cries out for more oxygen, new vessels grow in, but they are very fragile so they leak and produce destructive haemorrhages that leave fluid and protein deposits in the vitreous humour. In severe cases, matters progress to an even worse condition where excessive proliferation of the blood vessels causes deep bleeding. The scars that then form gradually pull the retina off the sclera altogether. Tractional retinal detachment follows and the eye is finished. So we must treat the ischaemic retinal tissues with lasers, and fortunately we can destroy the problematic part of the retina.

But this lands you with a dilemma. It's a bartering process – undertaking controlled destruction in order to keep some sight. So as to control the demand for oxygen, part of the retina is destroyed in the hope that the remaining blood vessels can provide a sufficient supply and the patient will keep the sight they still have.

An argon laser enables a surgeon to achieve much smaller burns compared with the xenon arc, though they may enlarge over a period of months or years. Sometimes our original burns are not sufficient, even though the surgeon may have done several hundreds or thousands. If that is the case, more will have to be done. This particular procedure does leave visual field defects about which patients may or may not be aware, which can mean the end of such activities as driving, but the remaining living cells are sufficient for a reasonable degree of vision. When extensive laser treatment is the only option, we always warn patients in advance about this possible consequence.

Other lasers such as the PASCAL laser (a trademark name) work on the same principle. Now the whole procedure becomes much faster, firing in patterns and achieving multiple burns simultaneously. This is a huge advantage, for doing 3,000 burns singly would be very labour intensive.

Lasers for refractive surgery

The excimer laser – which stands for excited dimer – was introduced in the 1980s and actually vaporises tissues atom by atom. The level of precision it can provide is remarkable. When Professor John Marshall developed the argon fluoride laser at St Thomas' Hospital in the mid-1980s, he produced a very famous slide of a human hair magnified by a scanning electron microscope. His laser then went on to cut grooves on the hair! By controlling laser energy very precisely, the cornea can be reshaped and a new optical effect produced. The short sight that I have had since childhood was transformed to normal sight by laser surgery in July 2002.

Next is the femtosecond laser – a name that reflects the time of its pulse. This, too, works very fast and can cut the cornea from within. Though the beam goes straight through the cornea it doesn't affect the top layer at all; rather, it creates a pocket within the layer. This supremely precise instrument is already being deployed extensively in laser refractive surgery, as a replacement for a mechanical blade called a microkeratome. Experimental cataract surgery is also being done with the femtosecond laser. The femtosecond laser remains hugely expensive and in most models, large in size. However, technology moves fast so miniaturisation and economy will soon arrive.

Lasers for treatment of glaucoma

Argon lasers can also be used to treat glaucoma, a condition characterised by raised eye pressure (it is not related to high blood pressure), damage to the optic nerve and later on tunnel vision. In the common form called open angle glaucoma, a contact lens with a mirror directs the laser light directly onto the angle of the eye. The angle is formed by where the back of the peripheral cornea meets the peripheral iris, and where the eye fluid aqueous humour is drained away. This drainage can be clogged up in glaucoma. By placing thermal burns in this area, the cells are rejuvenated and the pores in the angle are also opened by thermal contraction. Only half of the angle is treated, and the procedure has to be repeated from time to time. A more modern variant called selective laser trabeculoplasty (SLT) places larger, non-thermal, laser spots. This is said to be more gentle on the drainage angle.

In some glaucoma operations known as trabeculectomy, a pressure valve consisting of tiny holes that act like a trap door is created, and these open when the pressure is too high and allow the fluid to seep through. At the end of the operation stitches tie this valve down, but only lightly, for it has to lift a little to release fluid. If our sutures are applied too tightly, the fluid cannot pass and everything may seal together again. The argon laser or another thermal laser can be used to cut nylon stitches where these are used for a trabeculectomy procedure, thus relieving overly-tight stitching.

On the other hand, if they are too loose, then there is no difference in the pressure between the inside and the outside, so the eye goes soft and other complications set in. Thus in another variation, we use releasable sutures. The stitching is done, tied with a bow, which is left outside the field of operation and later released.

YAG laser treatment for narrow angle glaucoma is detailed below.

Laser treatment of ingrowing eyelashes

Thermal lasers can be used to annihilate the roots of aberrant eyelashes. When diseased or damaged, lashes may grow inwards, rub on the eye and be very irritating. Sometimes new, abnormal lashes can grow as a pathological response and cause abrasions on the eye surface, with potential for infection and consequent loss of vision. Lashes can be plucked out, but they will grow again. They can be removed by electrolysis in which, as in cosmetic surgery, an electric current is applied to the root in an attempt to kill it. This is only successful in two-thirds of cases. Lasering is another method, but still the lash can grow back. Usually, up to three treatment sessions are necessary to achieve complete success.

YAG laser

Last but not least is the YAG – Yttrium Aluminium Garnet – laser that produces photodisruption (microscopic atomic explosion), used for a complication of cataract surgery I researched earlier when I was based in Norwich. The posterior lens capsule is retained following cataract surgery to provide early support for the lens implant. Lens epithelial cells can grow underneath the implant onto the posterior capsule. The cells can become multilayered and form protein globules that obscure sight.

The YAG laser is focused carefully on the central part of the thickened posterior capsule. Two cuts are made, down and across, forming a cross. The four leaves fold away, revealing a clear central opening through which the patient can see again. It is important to focus carefully, otherwise the implant can be inadvertently lasered causing surface pits or even fracturing the implant. The opening has to be large enough so the surrounding thickened frill does not cause glare. However, there has to be sufficient remaining frill to continue to hold the implant in place. As the central posterior capsule has now folded away, new cells cannot grow into the area to obscure sight. YAG laser posterior capsulotomy is therefore a one-off treatment and rarely requires repeating.

The YAG laser can be used for problems other than posterior capsular thickening, such as those caused if the anterior chamber of the eye, where fluid strains away, is too shallow. Then the iris can go right up against the back of the cornea and block the chamber. The crystalline lens, the only organ that grows throughout life, can also add to the blockage.

The eye pressure can suddenly shoot very high and people can go blind within a few hours. They see rainbow coloured haloes, experience intense pain, feel sick and actually vomit. They can sometimes end up in casualty being assessed for what may be wrong with their stomach, when in fact all the symptoms derive from severe pain as their eye is stretched to the very extreme. So whenever there is acute eye pain, people should present to an eye surgeon immediately because the condition can then be reversed.

When using YAG laser photodisruption to release fluid, three successive pulses are directed at the peripheral iris very close together in time. The iris is punched, but before the laser pulse bounces back, another pulse comes in and then another. The iris is not a uniform structure but has ridges and valleys. So after asking the patient to keep still the surgeon selects a valley, as this is the thinnest part.

Everybody stops breathing; you focus accurately and then press the button. If the pulse goes through you see a gush of fluid along with the pigment from the back layer of the iris coming through like a waterfall. The hole you made may be tiny, but nevertheless the pressure is equalised for the flow of the fluid keeps it open. Surgically, you have to be extremely confident, though it's not the end of the world if you don't succeed the first time. The iris may be hit at some point and it can happen, although it is unlikely, that a blood vessel directly behind may be punctured. If that happens you press on the lens to increase the eye's pressure and stop the flow. Then the body's own coagulating mechanism clogs the vessel, and you either leave the procedure for another time or try somewhere else and find another valley. We still need to keep a 'beady eye' on all the holes to make certain they stay that way, because, just as in ear-piercing, the hole can become blocked again. These patients are monitored for the rest of their lives.

Whilst it is not possible to predict where the next development in lasers may be, we are certain that it is vitally important to increase their precision, their ease of use and drastically cut down their running and maintenance costs.

These machines cost from tens of thousands to several hundred thousand pounds each, so whether in the private or public sector, a high volume of patients has to be treated in order for them to be economically viable.

* * *

Age-related macular degeneration

Macular degeneration – a retinal problem and one of the most common forms of blindness in older people – affects more than 500,000 Britons and as people live longer, the numbers affected increase. This is no longer treated by laser.

The problem appears in two types, dry and wet. The dry type occurs because the eye can no longer deal with metabolic waste products. As a result, these are dumped in the middle of the retina and affect the central vision, compromising the ability to read and recognise people. The risk factors include smoking but diet, too, is very important. Given a choice between eating a lot of red meat or dark leafy vegetables and carrots, the patient should choose the vegetables. Dry macular degeneration tends to progress slowly but can transform into the wet type.

This is so called because fluid accumulates through leaky vessels breaching Bruch's membrane, and then blood vessels from the choroid come through. When this happens they can leak or bleed, and this produces the liquid. A major advance in treatment has been injections, right into the eye, of an anti-VEGF (anti-vascular endothelial growth factor) that cause the blood vessels to shrivel up and allow the patient to see. These injections are very expensive and often need to be repeated at regular intervals.

* * *

Another approach at the very cutting edge of science is not so much an external tool as drawing on the properties of our own cells. The best contemporary example involves stem cells and this is being tried for problems encountered both at the front of the eye and at the back.

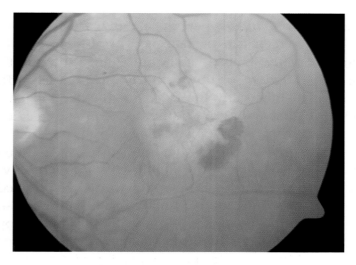

Fundus photo of wet type age-related macular degeneration.

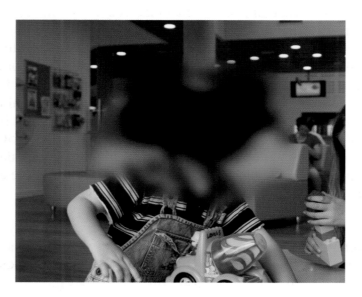

Macular degeneration gives rise to loss of central vision making reading and
recognising faces difficult or impossible.

121

Mention has already been made of corneal epithelial stem cells, which can be damaged by disease or injury. These live at the limbus, at the junction of the coloured part and the white of the eye. They are like seeds and provide daughter cells for covering the surface of the cornea, or the watch glass of the eye.

Stem cells capable of transforming into all sorts of tissues and organs are found in the bone marrow, peripheral blood and other areas in the adult body, although they are difficult to extract. It is also possible to trick differentiated cells to regress into more primitive stem cells (so-called 'turning the clock back', or induced pluripotent stem cells). Whilst it is possible to extract stem cells from early embryos, it is probably best to obtain them from the patient's own body. That way, the DNA is matched and there will be no immunological rejection. Extracting and using adult stem cells also means no ethical dilemma of having to sacrifice a potential life. Yet another possibility is to retrieve stem cells from the umbilical cord. These can be stored for later use, should the baby require stem cells for therapy later in life.

The beauty of stem cells is their ability to regenerate and repair tissues and organs. In terms of eye treatment, delivery of stem cells is often difficult. In the case of retinal disease, such as age-related macular degeneration, inherited retinal dystrophies, and diabetic retinopathy, the cells will have to be placed through a surgical operation.

Gene therapy is another cutting edge technology for treatment of disease, but much of it is experimental. In somatic gene therapy, a missing or defective gene is replaced with the help of a vector, usually a virus. Work is also being done on in situ production of anti-VEGF using gene therapy, so as to avoid the requirement of repeated injections of anti-VEGF agents for treatment of wet age-related macular degeneration.

Finally, if the eye and/or optic nerve should fail altogether, artificial vision technology could be called upon. Current devices do not yet work adequately, and are experimental. These systems consist essentially of a camera with electrical outputs connected to the visual cortex.

Patients seeking new technology for treatment of their eye problems should be aware that the majority of new technology is experimental, may not work, and carries risks. Anything brand new is necessarily not fully proven and may not withstand the test of time.

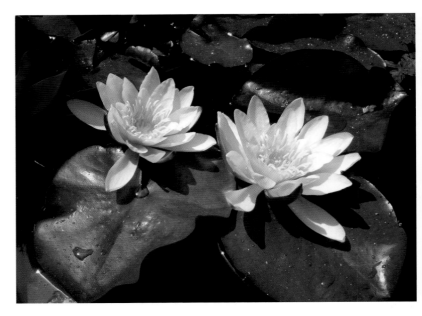

Water lilies in the pond of our front garden in Hove.

9

Wider Outlooks

The life of a consultant does not only consist of diagnosing, operating and treating but also training the next generation. At the moment, trainees come to the Sussex Eye Hospital for just one year and rotate through different consultants every four months. You don't get to know them and they don't get to know you. I may be old-fashioned but I am very keen on learning by apprenticeship; this would entail staying at the same place for perhaps two years and rotating every six months.

Trainees are not here only to learn a few diagnostic, clinical and surgical skills. If you want to craft a complete doctor you need much more time, for it's not just a technical exercise but rather it encompasses a holistic approach to the patient. Ideally it should be as in ancient Greek times, when a young person going through school learnt not just the subject, but the philosophy and approach to life.

This is how it was in my day. You would join a hospital and stay for a long period. At Moorfields it was always one-on-one – consultant and trainee – rotating every six months. Recently everything has changed; the process is more fragmented with a curriculum-based approach in a programme designed to run over many years. The trainee goes to a different place, group or person, and every time is supposed to learn one small part of the total curriculum. This new system didn't happen arbitrarily; there were reasons for changing. One was so the entire curriculum would be covered, whereas previously the trainee would be exposed to fewer areas so there were gaps in one's medical knowledge. However, I believe this doesn't matter all that much, because an important focus within medicine is to act within your own capabilities and refer to others if you need help.

By the time trainees have finished these days, they may have learnt all the technical skills, but still haven't done a proper apprenticeship. Indeed, there are few countries that stick to the old ways. The change from the traditional apprenticeship to a more structured, vocational – but perhaps also a more superficial – system has also taken place in countries such as Australia, which emulated the British approach to health care professional training. These changes have made a one-on-one, year-long fellowship even more important, for it is more of an apprenticeship model, a kind of finishing school taken at the end of training.

Different trainers have different methods and opinions. When I have a new trainee they do no operating for the first week, even if they are very experienced, because I want them to observe me working and to familiarise themselves with the environment before they start. When starting in a totally new environment, your results during the first few weeks are bound to be compromised. I see that year after year, whenever a new crop of doctors comes along. The equipment, the instruments and the people they must relate to are all different. They may have just moved, or be commuting by an unfamiliar route and all such factors can overwhelm the brain. I am usually very gentle and after some weeks they are back to their usual operating ability.

Before I let my trainees loose, I want to get to know them better and understand their personalities. Of course, they are never let entirely loose to begin with, for I watch on the monitors. Deciding when the trainee can start on his or her own is a critical moment, just like sending a pilot solo for the first time. Before this can happen we need to have frequent conversations, until I am convinced that even though they have observed me many times, they really do have a genuine grasp of what needs to be done during an operation.

It is often said that there are three stages to learning surgery; first you have to learn how to do it; next you learn when to do it; finally, you learn when not to do it. You have to be able to say no; one should think twice before taking on a seemingly hopeless case when the patient has unrealistic expectations of success. There are several ways a trainee surgeon can build both skill and confidence. Nowadays young people never do the whole operation, but go as far as they can and if they get anxious, or the procedure is not going well, their mentor takes over. Another method is to allow them to do the last part of an operation – the stitching for example – rather than the first part, because if this does not go well, matters would be even more difficult by the time the consultant takes over. The wound might not be perfect; indeed it might be leaky. It is the same when a new presenter fronts a television series. The last episode to be broadcast is filmed first, so by the time the first one to be broadcast is filmed, the presenter has the skills and confidence and immediately makes a good impression.

Of course, trainees practise constantly, initially on model eyes made of wax or plastic. A cataract operation can be divided into many stages, so they will practise the same part over and over and sometimes do this on 'pretend' eyes in the wet lab, or even on the eyes of dead animals. Although these never feel the same as human eyes, nowadays all trainees must pass an obligatory microsurgical course before they are allowed to cut a human eye. This is in great contrast to my experience, for when I started, I was more or less allowed to do the whole operation in one go.

Another important aspect in training the next generation of surgeons is exposing them to a number of teachers so as to get different experiences in different subspecialties. However, in the current system they are moving on too frequently; when people move quickly they never settle and do not really learn about long-term evolution of the condition or disease. They need to watch and monitor the patients for far longer periods, otherwise they just learn technique but not doctoring. I think each person should stay in the same place for two years and then move on to another place for a further two. Within those periods they could still be attached to different teachers, either separately or concurrently.

Another essential quality is self-confidence, yet while a great deal of this comes from learning, training and experience, it is generally felt that people who decide to become surgeons simply must have plenty before they start. My personal opinion – though I admit this may be biased – is that compared to general or orthopaedic surgeons, who really think they can do it all, eye surgeons are far more introspective and always have some self-doubt – not a bad thing. This is triggered in part by the very nature of the small, complex organ that they deal with. The scale is so small and there is so little margin for error, that the eye forces you to face your own limitations.

Yet still there's much more to one's learning process than technique and repetitive procedures. The dimensions of current medical practice and the issues that impact upon it are becoming more varied and difficult, with persistent ethical overtones. For example, our founder, James Pickford, didn't believe in vivisection and certainly would not have tolerated any human experimentation. However, during the nineteenth century the need for some form of animal experimentation became evident, pioneered by the famous French physiologist, Claude Bernard, so attitudes changed gradually.

If we could do everything we need to do with just tissue cultures or models and use only donated human eye tissue for research, this would have two benefits; no animals would be used and the results would apply straight away to human disease. But we are not yet in this situation. My view is that while it is probably necessary to do some animal experimentation, this *must* be reduced to an absolute minimum.

Another aspect a young surgeon must weigh up is the value and importance of evidence-based medicine. Some of what we do was handed down to us by our teachers as accepted practice because 'this is what we've been doing for years', with no basis in evidence. Actually, until proper scientific experiments with clinical trials came in, this was all that medicine was.

Then randomised clinical trials came in and without them, approval for therapies is not given. OOKP provided a fine example of how the challenge could prove highly complex, for it was a struggle to get the procedure approved at all. The evidence base was highly unusual, to say the least, and at the beginning all we could produce was the fact that the operation had been going on in Italy for thirty to forty years, and if nothing was done patients remained blind. Was that good enough evidence, or not? Initially the answer was no. But eventually the authorities came round to understanding that you *cannot* experiment in such situations, because we knew that nothing else would work. Nor could we do a random clinical trial since the incidence of the disease is so low – five patients a year – that it is impossible to expect the results to be statistically valid. Would it be ethical to divide patients into two groups and give one OOKP and the second another treatment that you knew would fail?

There is another factor. Crucial though randomised controlled trials are, even the best ones have their limitations. If there is something – such as OOKP – that is obviously better than any alternative, then not only can you not go through a clinical trial, but you probably don't need to. Indeed there have been trials where the results are coming through loud and clear and are of such statistical significance that the trial is stopped, since it becomes unethical not to treat the control group at that point. Recently, Memorial Sloan-Kettering Cancer Center in New York announced success with a new drug that was yielding excellent results for the treatment of melanoma, a deadly skin disease. The drug worked by controlling the gene that triggers the metastasis, the process whereby a cancer cell leaves the tumour and is carried around the body where it starts a tumour in another organ. The results were so spectacularly good that the trial was halted and everyone treated.

In addition to everything else, students must learn that there are classes of evidence that have existed for a long time. The top class in the Oxford scale is meta-analysis of randomised control trials while the lowest is someone's professional opinion. Yet sometimes this actually counts for a lot and one must always remember that there is art in medicine as well as science. A trainee will soon come to realise that sometimes we have very little time to make a decision, especially in a surgical situation. Then you have to weigh up matters based on your own experience, either from what you've read, or what others have told you, or what you've learnt in your training, and just meld everything together. We call this 'fuzzy logic'. Since some people are blessed with the ability to do the right thing at the right time in a clinical situation, their 'fuzzy logic' becomes 'clinical acumen'. It is difficult to explain and though it can be passed on by an apprenticeship, it cannot readily be passed on by encountering clinical problems in many small curriculum modules over a short period of time.

Fuzzy logic, or rather clinical acumen, isn't just intuition; it is compounded of judgement that derives from experience, knowledge and understanding while simultaneously weighing up probabilities. Sometimes you have to make a highly complex decision in an incredibly short space of time. People with manifold problems can seek the help of a therapist over the long term, but in a critical surgical situation there is no time. If something does go wrong and a patient is angry or later decides to sue, then you have to go back and dissect your own thought process before instructing your solicitor and appearing in court.

A common way around such problems is to practise defensive medicine and consider that one might end up in court before doing anything. When that route is taken, too many tests are ordered and, as we see in the United States, medical practice becomes very costly both for the patient and for society. There has to be a balance. This is one reason why nowadays we have many presentations of difficult and challenging cases in our professional meetings to get people really thinking.

Yet even in routine work such as cataract surgery one must constantly challenge oneself. The procedure may be routine but it touches many lives. I do not allow anyone in my team to think of the operation as 'just another cataract', for it is the eye, sight and life of a fellow human being. I constantly remind them that every single part of each consultation and operation is unique to the patient – not only with regard to the person but to the eyes too. Before we start, we plan the surgery carefully, take consent and make clear to the patient just what can be achieved. Then the operation itself becomes like a precise military exercise, a matter of execution that you carry out to the best of your abilities.

On the other hand, a touch of the exotic is also important for us all, whether consultants or trainees. The exotic focuses your mind and keeps it active. Not only is there a practical advantage in being expert at a particular task, but peer recognition also follows and that allows you to talk to people of equal standing at other institutions. You can question and learn from them. I can call upon such people and because they know I am a genuine person who does valuable work, they take me seriously. This has been very important for my own development and how I provide patient care.

Moreover, by doing the exotic work as well as the routine, you place your hospital in a higher position and this attracts higher calibre staff, whether nursing, administrative or trainees. Then patient care will improve. Good trainees may come back to join the staff, or create a new department.

Equally it must be remembered that trainees train their trainers too, not only because they have been to other hospitals and made new observations, but because they have fresh, young minds. They ask difficult questions which their teacher has to answer. This is a really important two-way process in which everyone stands to gain. Such revitalisation is important for all consultants.

Someone once said that the problem of scientific old age is not hardening of the arteries, so much as hardening of the categories, when you think purely inside your own personal boundaries. As time goes by, your own categories become entrenched or misguided. The joy and importance of young people is that they not only challenge you, but are also thinking outside the categories. One must be flexible enough to know when things have changed and not be too dogmatic.

However, there are sometimes exacting situations that no-one has dealt with before. Then I recognise that it is going to be difficult, but it is within my field. Though challenging, I will work out a strategy, thinking through from the basics and using different methods and tools. On that basis I have devised a number of new techniques and instruments. These include implanting two rigid intra-ocular lenses at the same time to make up the necessary optical power. We call that dual in the bag piggyback PMMA lens implants! Another is the two point fixation forceps, which allow a better grasp of the eye during surgery. A third is a redesigned optical cylinder for OOKP surgery that allows a wider visual field. To do this you have to have a clear mind. A new operation may finally only take an hour or so, but can take dozens of hours to plan,

- Improved optical cylinder designs for artificial cornea to improve clarity and field of view.
- A laboratory model for preliminary biological screening of potential keratoprosthetic biomaterials.
- Employing electron beam tomography to assess osteo-odonto-keratoprosthesis laminar dimensions.
- Automated volumetric assessment of osteo-odonto-keratoprostheses.
- The Norwich *in vitro* model for studying posterior capsular opacification following cataract surgery.
- Discovery of ability of human lens epithelial cell to survive and proliferate in a protein free culture medium.
- Discovery of the ability of thapsigargin to inhibit human lens epithelial cell growth.
- Two point fixation forceps for corneal sections in cataract surgery.
- Using iris retraction hooks for cataract surgery in patients with iridoschisis.
- Using multiple capsular tension rings for prevention of capsular contraction syndrome following cataract surgery.
- Primary polypseudophakia for cataract surgery in long sighted eyes using two PMMA intraocular lens implants within the lens capsular bag.
- Description of a safe protocol for operating on both eyes at the same sitting for cataract surgery.
- 'Cataract Surgery by Appointment'.
- 'Bowl and Snail' technique for soft cataracts.
- Description of an algorithm to enhance communication with hearing impaired patients during cataract surgery.
- Description of strategic use of a yellow blue-blocking implant and one eye and a clear lens implant in the other to reduce the risk of progression of macular degeneration.
- 'Black on Clear' dual in the bag opaque and clear intraocular lenses to relieve intractable double vision.
- Scanning electron microscopic study of monofilament nylon knots to confirm superiority of the 2-1-1 reef knot.
- Harvesting autologous conjunctiva from the lower part of the globe for primary pterygium surgery.
- Experimental ciliary tissue transplantation.
- The 'Liu position' for safe placement of retrobulbar local anaesthesia.
- The '2+1' anaesthesia technique for patients undergoing cataract surgery.

Some innovations and inventions by the author and his collaborators especially when what you propose has never been done before.

I know that in order to do all this – teach, supervise, practise and carry out research – I need to regularly renew my mental capacity. I am much refreshed by exercising regularly, massage, collecting paintings, travel, meditating and old-fashioned contemplation.

One final challenge a young practitioner must face is extremely sensitive, for this relates to the dynamics between young and old. A point finally comes when one is no longer as sharp as before. Each person has a natural ceiling of performance that can be nurtured through training, and that ceiling can be maintained through having a healthy mind and body. Surgeons usually have a pretty inflated opinion of themselves, which is not necessarily bad, as decisive actions often have to be taken. Some will have more insight than others. Theatre scrub nurses and anaesthetists are extremely good at recognising the skill and judgement of surgeons. If you ever need a recommendation, ask them!

The General Medical Council insists that if necessary, everyone should be a whistle-blower. All of us are supposed to raise concern if anyone, even a close colleague, is clearly underperforming. If I know that something is amiss and don't blow the whistle, then my own medical registration is genuinely at risk. This provokes a difficult ethical challenge for if there are interpersonal problems, false accusations may be raised and cause a heap of difficulties. This applies not just to surgery but also to the whole business of doctoring. When do you say to a colleague that he is now sub-standard? And just where do you draw the line? These are questions and challenges that cannot be ignored.

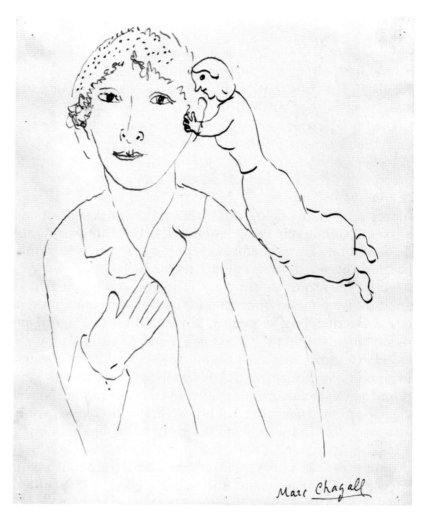

La voix du Coeur. Artist: Marc Chagall.
Chagall®/© ADAGP, Paris and DACS, London 2011.

10

Full Circle

In 2007, eleven years after I became a consultant at the Sussex Eye Hospital, we celebrated the 175th anniversary of its founding, an occasion for celebration and reflection, both institutional and personal.

James Pickford would hardly recognise the place, so great is the volume of our work and so wide our international connections. However, he would be most gratified to see that the Pickford Ward still remains, though now we also have a few single rooms, a day case room and a partitioned mixed ward. Each year we do between 3,000 and 4,000 cataract operations, see 50,000 outpatients, treat 10,000 to 15,000 ophthalmic accident and emergency episodes, as well as handling several thousand orthoptic appointments.

Our staff, who serve outpatients, accidents and emergencies, the wards and the theatre, number over 100 people and include 7 full-time consultants as well as managers, matrons, nurses, technicians and clerical staff. Our budget runs into millions of pounds a year.

I was the convenor for the celebrations held on 23rd November 2007 and preparations took a year. Unlike 1930,

137

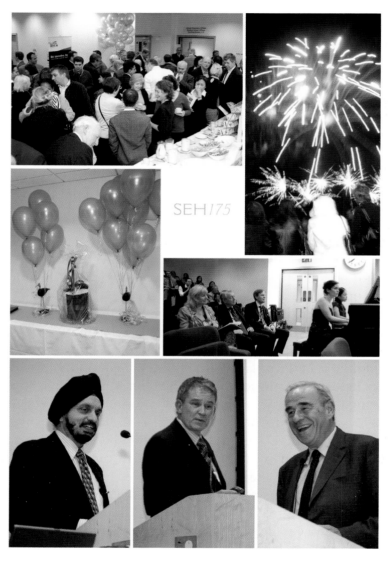

Clockwise from top left: Tea break; Fireworks at the seafront; Piano recital; Richard Keeler, Bruce McLeod; Professor Harminder Dua; 175th birthday cake flanked by blue and silver balloons.

138

the function was limited to one day, not three, and while no ambassadors – French or otherwise – were present, over 200 delegates came from all over the world. Though we had neither tableaux nor pageants, we mounted a splendid evening of entertainment, preceded during the day by a series of short talks in an auditorium decorated with 350 balloons, half of them silver and half blue. Our duality of purpose, to serve patients and advance ophthalmology, both research and teaching, determined our choice of colours.

Silver was a statement about the level of service we give to our patients. Blue, like the sky, summed up the infinity of our aspirations, for one day we hope to have a royal patron and so become the Royal Sussex Eye Hospital. This is not an unrealistic ambition as the three local hospitals that make up the Brighton and Sussex University Hospitals NHS Trust are already favoured. These are our nextdoor neighbours – the Royal Sussex County Hospital, the Royal Alexandra Hospital for Children and the Princess Royal Hospital in Haywards Heath.

Scientists may sometimes be portrayed as dry as dust, but during our celebrations we showed humour and imagination, especially in the titles of our lectures: 'Searching for the Magic Potion', a survey of effective treatments for glaucoma, given by Fiona O'Sullivan; 'Going Up To Hogwarts', about the nursing courses, delivered by Sister Gaynor Paul, our lead nurse in Outpatient and Casualty; 'Aladdin's Cave', delivered by Richard Keeler, the Curator of the Royal College of Ophthalmology Museum, that covered fascinating examples of early instruments, books and potions; 'Alice In Wonderland – Seeing Things', delivered by Sarah Vickers, who highlighted neuro-ophthalmological conditions that produce visual hallucinations. My own presentation, 'Dark They Were and Golden Eyed', focused on the hospital's research programmes and the process by which an immigrant – myself – became totally assimilated into British society.

Our evening diversions included a piano recital and the eighteenth Sussex Eye Hospital Endowment Lecture, 'The Eye of the Beholder', given by Professor Harminder Singh Dua. This was a fascinating account of the varied and wonderful eyes that are found in different animals. Our speaker was given our most grateful thanks and a specially-commissioned watercolour of the hospital by Bill Black-shaw, Honorary Member of the Royal Watercolour Society (HRH The Prince of Wales is also an Honorary Member). [The painting appears on the front of this book's jacket.] A spectacular firework display on the beach front came next, followed by a buffet supper, during which, along with breakfast at the Grand Hotel next morning, everyone had time to catch up, reminisce and wallow in nostalgia.

One thing has always been missing from all celebrations whenever held: a picture of James Pickford. Not one single portrait, sketch, or photograph of our founder has ever been discovered, though not for want of trying. All likely sources have been tapped, including the archives of the Regimental Footguards and the Sussex Family History Association. Pickford had no grandchildren and though photography had been invented before he died, there are neither public nor family documents to help us.

We celebrated other people and other legacies too. The Brighton Society for the Blind, once fondly called The Lantern, now The Sussex Lantern, whose previous head-quarters were at William Moon Lodge, is one of many lasting triumphs of William Moon, whose work paralleled that of Pickford. Close links with the Sussex Eye Hospital were revived in the last two decades of the twentieth century as Gloria Wright, who has worked for the society since 1987, recalls. In February 1999 she became director, a post she held until 2004 when she became secretary and trustee. Shortly after she joined, the society was able to move out of two small rooms in a home for people with Alzheimer's disease to new headquarters in the large Claremont Church Hall, and had in no time at all raised the £27,000 needed for major renovations. The administrative offices were placed upstairs, the day centre and rehabilitation centre were downstairs. They started with just twenty staff and clients, but by Christmas the same year, one hundred and twenty people sat down for the party.

The money came mainly from trusts, but also from ordinary people, who in those days would happily donate £100 or £1,500. The president of the society was Sir John Wilson, an unsung but unstinting supporter. He lost his sight at the age of twelve following an accident in his school's chemistry laboratory. Sir John's main concern was to bring eye care within the reach of deprived communities, and his work was to have a profound impact on the lives of millions of people in many of the poorest countries in the world.

In 1950, Sir John founded Sight Savers International, formerly known as the Royal Commonwealth Society for the Blind, and led the organisation for more than thirty years. His genius was innovation: he established many of the essential elements underpinning eye care services in developing countries; he was instrumental in revealing the scale of world blindness, the first conservative estimate being 15 million people, and inspired the global collaboration essential to tackling human suffering on this huge scale.

In the 1920s, when the Norma Lees Fund provided money for medical help, links with the hospital's doctors had been strong. Seventy years later the society felt that help for those losing their sight could be best met by providing immediate contact and a counselling service. They set up an information desk with two nursing sisters right in the Eye Hospital, the first ever in Britain. Soon many referrals came in and home visiting started.

The twenty-first century brings fresh demands. Gloria Wright believes that since such wonderful treatment is now available for eye conditions, the need for a day centre has diminished. When she first joined the Brighton Society for the Blind, every phone call was about cataracts and most patients felt they should have an operation immediately. Nurses at the Eye Hospital's information desk could explain to people why they had to wait until the eye was ready, and supported them through the waiting period.

Though they still get referrals from the Eye Hospital, these are for many different conditions for which a range of superb treatments and operations are now available. The change in pattern of referral has resulted from the great success with cataract surgery, new treatments for macular degeneration and the existence of laser surgery to treat other eye problems. On the educational side, too, there have been vast improvements from the way people are taught at school about their eyes, to the quality of general health and the increased level of support in the community. All this has had an amazing impact on eye care.

Recently, the society has moved into a new purpose-built centre in Keymer near Hassocks, West Sussex. Major funds were raised yet again, since they wanted the property to be sustainable and financially easy to run. Part of the building provides holiday and leisure facilities for the disabled and the blind. They would like to add an educational section because they know that whatever the disability – blindness, partial sight or something quite different – it is important for people to be able to communicate.

Looking back over the 175 years of remarkable history, the successes are not only a wonderful testament to the pioneers such as Pickford and Moon, but also to the town of Brighton, its people and society. From the very beginning when it blossomed into a fashionable seaside town, the poor, the disabled and the sick have never been forgotten.

The city is also home to the St Dunstan's centre. Founded 96 years ago by Arthur Pearson, visually impaired owner of the *Daily Express*, St Dunstan's has remained true to its original mission to help blind ex-servicemen and women lead independent and fulfilling lives. Today St Dunstan's gives invaluable physical and emotional support to thousands of blind and visually impaired ex-servicemen and women with its unique expertise, experience and comprehensive range of services. The charity is there for its beneficiaries for as long as they need, helping them to adjust to their loss of sight and learn new skills – and its support lasts a lifetime, helping families too, as they adjust to their changing needs.

* * *

Brighton continues to support the blind and Rayner continues to flourish, recently receiving the Queen's Award for Enterprise in International Trade for their intraocular lenses. Whilst these lenses are still occasionally made from the same plastic material – Perspex – used by Sir Harold

Ridley after World War Two, there is a drawback. It is a rigid material and getting it into the eye is as difficult as putting a fat letter through a slim letterbox. During the 1980s and 1990s, surgeons began to complain that while they needed only a small incision to liquefy and vacuum out a cataract, they then had to increase the incision by another 5 mm just to get the lens in. The manufacturers were challenged; make smaller, foldable lenses, though not too small because there is an optimum size for optical function. True to form, Rayner and others came up with different materials that could fold, or be compressed, and then injected into the eye through a keyhole wound.

The instrument used is about the size of a small pen; the mechanism is similar in action to a hypodermic needle and a syringe. The plunger is depressed and the lens pushed through a small nozzle into the eye. Once in place in the capsule, it unfolds in position. Rayner have been most innovative and, working closely with surgeons, continue to develop new types of intraocular lenses. One such invention is an implant with an inbuilt prism for use in eyes with macular degeneration, so the focused image is directed to adjacent healthy retina. Another is a supplementary (piggyback) implant which can be inserted to fine tune unexpected refractive outcome following cataract surgery. One form of this piggyback implant can also add multifocality, enabling patients to see both distance and near without glasses.

* * *

In all kinds of ways we have come full circle. Our 175th anniversary was a time to reflect on the development of our profession, and in the last few years I have been reflecting on my own career. In the British medical field,

FULL CIRCLE

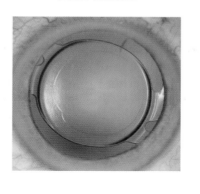

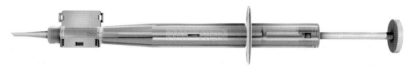

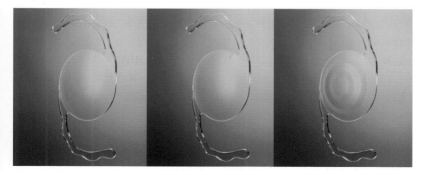

Top: Rayner aspheric intraocular lens within the lens capsular bag against red reflex showing perfect clarity and centration.
Middle: Rayner intraocular lens injector. The lens implant is placed in the cartridge on the left. The soft blue sponge advances the lens through the funnelled tip. The lens implant folds itself through the tip, enters the eye through a keyhole wound, and gently unfolds to its original shape and size once inside the eye.
Bottom: The innovative Rayner Sulcoflex family of supplementary intraocular lenses.
Images courtesy of Rayner Intraocular Lenses Limited.

people tend to divide the thirty-odd years of professional life, following ten of training, into three phases: first, you establish yourself; then you slow down a little, perhaps teach more and operate less; finally, during the last five to ten years, management tasks predominate or consultancy work for one of the royal medical colleges or the government.

After fifteen years as a consultant, I am midway through the second phase and have another fifteen years or so to go. Having looked back at my career thus far, I have clear ideas about what I would like to achieve in the future. First of all, I will continue research into the delivery and safety of cataract surgery, including operating on both eyes at the same sitting. I would like to understand why a small number of patients are dissatisfied with cataract surgery in order to eliminate this problem. Second, I will continue to develop the Sussex Eye Hospital as the national referral centre for OOKP surgery. In addition to the OOKP, I want to provide a whole range of artificial corneae, a process that has already started. We now offer the Pintucci device, made of plastic and Dacron, as well as the device developed at Harvard made of plastic and titanium. The research and clinical work takes me all over the world to teach and demonstrate surgery, as well as to learn from others.

I am lucky in what I do and where I do it. Ophthalmology remains my abiding passion. The eyes certainly have it, but so too do Brighton and Hove, and the Sussex Eye Hospital.

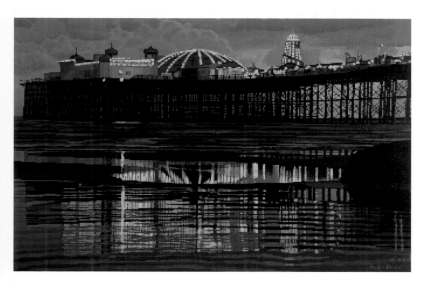

Water colour of the Palace Pier (now Brighton Pier) by Philip Dunn.

Afterword

In our youth, while we unwittingly create history we loathe reading it. As we mature we look back, reflect, absorb and learn from history as we plan for the future. When we prepare to fade away into history, we will have done well if we leave behind an imprint that others can learn from and be inspired by. In this book, Christopher Liu, a distinguished ophthalmologist who has contributed much to British ophthalmology, reflects on the first half of his consultant career as he plans for the second, well on course towards leaving a lasting impression.

Harminder S Dua MBBS, DO, DO(Lond.), MS, MNAMS, FRCS, PRCOphth., FEBO, MD, PhD

Chair and Professor of Ophthalmology, University of Nottingham
President, Royal College of Ophthalmologists, UK
President, European Society of Cornea and Ocular Surface Disease Specialists (EuCornea)
President, European Association for Vision and Eye Research Foundation (EVER*f*)
Editor-in-chief, *British Journal of Ophthalmology*
Past President, European Association for Vision and Eye Research (EVER)

Further Reading

For information about **ophthalmia and the origin of eye hospitals** see:

Auden, Rita R, *A Hunterian Pupil: Sir William Blizard and The London Hospital*
Annals of the Royal College of Surgeons of England, vol.60, pages 345–349, 1978

Cantlie, Lt Gen Sir Neil, *A History of the Army Medical Department,* vol.I, Churchill Livingstone, Edinburgh & London, 1974

Marmion, V J, *The Origin of Eye Hospitals* British Journal of Ophthalmology, 89(11) 1396–1397. November 2005

De Sousa, M Leonor Machado, *English Surgery and Portugal* Journal of The Royal Society of Medicine, vol.78, pages 239–245. March 1985

Vetch, John, *An Account of the Ophthalmia which has Appeared in England since the Return of the British Army from Egypt* Longman, Hurst, Rees & Orme, London 1807

For information about **James Pickford**

The Medical Directory 1865
Obituary Brighton Gazette, 21st January 1875
Obituary Brighton Herald, 23rd January 1875
Special Library & Archives in Library and Historic Collections, Kings College, University of Aberdeen. *www.abdn. ac.uk/historic*

For information about **William Moon**

Alphabets and Literature for the Blind Casey Wood's Encyclopaedia, vol. XVI, p. 259-261

Perks, Joy Jennings, *The House of William Moon* publication pending. Sussex Lantern.

For information about **the Sussex Eye Hospital**

East Sussex Record Office: National Health Service: Brighton District Health Authority [HB/1–HB/94]
   HB/57, 171 SEH 1832
   HB/57 1927, 1946
   HB/96 Plans 1933

Howlett & Clark of Brighton, solicitors
   HOW/25 1800-1900, correspondence, receipts, annual reports, SEH
   HOW/26 1800-1900   "   "
   HOW/67/7 1909-1934   plans of intended buildings, SEH
   HOW/108/3 1846-1901   buildings, alterations, correspondence, minutes and Brighton History Centre: re

book collection. Annual Reports for 1875, 1883, 1891, 1893.

The Sussex Eye Hospital The Nursing Mirror & Midwives Journal, September 27th 1930, p.523-4

The Sussex Eye Hospital, 175th Anniversary Celebrations Eye News, Feb/Mar 2008, p. 69-70

Keeler, Richard, *175th Anniversary of the Sussex Eye Hospital* Museum Piece of College News. Quarterly Bulletin of The Royal College of Ophthalmologists, Autumn 200, p. 7

Laust, L W, *The Development of the Hospitals in Brighton & Hove* Royal Society of Medicine, vol.65, p. 221-226, February 1972

Other topics:

Barraquer, Joaquín, *Evolution of Cataract Surgery: Past, Present and Future* Anales del Instituto Barraquer, vol. xxxviii, num.1-2, p.71

Ching, Frank, *The Li Dynasty: Hong Kong Aristocrats,* Oxford University Press, 1999

Trevor-Roper, Patrick, *The World Through Blunted Sight* Souvenir Press, 1997